LEARNING TO I
MULTIPLE SC

DR ROBERT POVEY is an Educational Psychologist
and lecturer at Christ Church College, Canterbury. Dr
Povey has published various scientific papers and books.
He was elected to a Fellowship of the British Psychological Society in 1977. He is the husband of an MS
sufferer, and is a founder member of the Canterbury and
District branch of the Multiple Sclerosis Society.

ROBIN DOWIE is a Senior Research Fellow at the
British Postgraduate Medical Federation, University of
London. She has written a number of publications, and
was Secretary of the Canterbury and District branch of
the Multiple Sclerosis Society from 1976 to 1979.

GILLIAN PRETT is a lecturer in English Literature
and Communications at Canterbury College of Tech-
nology. She has been a committee member of the
Canterbury and District branch of the Multiple Sclerosis
Society since 1976 and was its secretary from 1979 to
1981. In 1981 she was a founder member of the
Association for the Independence of the Disabled, and
is its Vice Chairman.

Overcoming Common Problems Series

The ABC of Eating
Coping with anorexia, bulimia and
compulsive eating
JOY MELVILLE

An A–Z of Alternative Medicine
BRENT Q. HAFEN AND KATHRYN J.
FRANDSEN

Arthritis
Is your suffering really necessary?
DR WILLIAM FOX

Being the Boss
STEPHEN FITZSIMON

Birth Over Thirty
SHEILA KITZINGER

Body Language
How to read others' thoughts by their gestures
ALLAN PEASE

Bodypower
DR VERNON COLEMAN

Calm Down
How to cope with frustration and anger
DR PAUL HAUCK

Comfort for Depression
JANET HORWOOD

Common Childhood Illnesses
DR PATRICIA GILBERT

Complete Public Speaker
GYLES BRANDRETH

Coping with Anxiety and Depression
SHIRLEY TRICKETT

Coping with Depression and Elation
DR PATRICK McKEON

Coping with Stress
DR GEORGIA WITKIN-LANOIL

Coping with Suicide
DR DONALD SCOTT

Coping with Thrush
CAROLINE CLAYTON

Coping Successfully with Your Child's Asthma
DR PAUL CARSON

Coping Successfully with Your Child's Skin Problems
DR PAUL CARSON

Coping Successfully with Your Hyperactive Child
DR PAUL CARSON

Coping Successfully with Your Irritable Bowel
ROSEMARY NICOL

Curing Arthritis Cookbook
MARGARET HILLS

Curing Arthritis – The Drug-free Way
MARGARET HILLS

Curing Coughs, Colds and Flu – the Drug-free Way
MARGARET HILLS

Curing Illness – The Drug-free Way
MARGARET HILLS

Depression
DR PAUL HAUCK

Divorce and Separation
ANGELA WILLANS

The Dr Moerman Cancer Diet
RUTH JOCHEMS

The Epilepsy Handbook
SHELAGH McGOVERN

Everything You Need to Know about Adoption
MAGGIE JONES

Everything You Need to Know about Contact Lenses
DR ROBERT YOUNGSON

Everything You Need to Know about Your Eyes
DR ROBERT YOUNGSON

Everything You Need to Know about the Pill
WENDY COOPER AND TOM SMITH

Everything You Need to Know about Shingles
DR ROBERT YOUNGSON

Family First Aid and Emergency Handbook
DR ANDREW STANWAY

Feverfew
A traditional herbal remedy for migraine and arthritis
DR STEWART JOHNSON

Fight Your Phobia and Win
DAVID LEWIS

Overcoming Common Problems Series

Flying Without Fear
TESSA DUCKWORTH AND DAVID
MILLER

Goodbye Backache
DR DAVID IMRIE WITH COLLEEN
DIMSON

Good Publicity Guide
REGINALD PEPLOW

Helping Children Cope with Divorce
ROSEMARY WELLS

Helping Children Cope with Grief
ROSEMARY WELLS

How to Be Your Own Best Friend
DR PAUL HAUCK

How to Control your Drinking
DRS W. MILLER AND R. MUNOZ

How to Cope with Stress
DR PETER TYRER

How to Cope with your Child's Allergies
DR PAUL CARSON

How to Cope with your Nerves
DR TONY LAKE

How to Cope with Tinnitus and Hearing Loss
DR ROBERT YOUNGSON

How to Cure Your Ulcer
ANNE CHARLISH AND DR BRIAN
GAZZARD

How to Do What You Want to Do
DR PAUL HAUCK

How to Enjoy Your Old Age
DR B. F. SKINNER AND M. E.
VAUGHAN

How to Improve Your Confidence
DR KENNETH HAMBLY

How to Interview and Be Interviewed
MICHELE BROWN AND
GYLES BRANDRETH

How to Love a Difficult Man
NANCY GOOD

How to Love and be Loved
DR PAUL HAUCK

How to Make Successful Decisions
ALISON HARDINGHAM

How to Pass Your Driving Test
DONALD RIDLAND

How to Say No to Alcohol
KEITH McNEILL

How to Sleep Better
DR PETER TYRER

How to Stand up for Yourself
DR PAUL HAUCK

How to Start a Conversation and Make Friends
DON GABOR

How to Stop Feeling Guilty
DR VERNON COLEMAN

How to Stop Smoking
GEORGE TARGET

How to Stop Taking Tranquillisers
DR PETER TYRER

Hysterectomy
SUZIE HAYMAN

If Your Child is Diabetic
JOANNE ELLIOTT

Jealousy
DR PAUL HAUCK

Learning to Live with Multiple Sclerosis
DR ROBERT POVEY, ROBIN DOWIE
AND GILLIAN PRETT

Living Alone – A Womans Guide
LIZ McNEILL TAYLOR

Living with Grief
DR TONY LAKE

Living Through Personal Crisis
ANN KAISER STEARNS

Living with High Blood Pressure
DR TOM SMITH

Loneliness
DR TONY LAKE

Making Marriage Work
DR PAUL HAUCK

Overcoming Common Problems Series

Overcoming Common Problems

LEARNING TO LIVE WITH MULTIPLE SCLEROSIS

Dr Robert Povey, Robin Dowie
and Gillian Prett

Foreword by Professor Bryan Matthews
Illustrations by Keith Lovet Watson

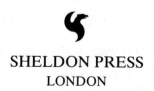

SHELDON PRESS
LONDON

First published in 1981 by the Multiple Sclerosis
Society of Great Britain and Northern Ireland

Revised edition published in Great Britain in 1986
by Sheldon Press, SPCK, Marylebone Road, London NW1 4DU

Second impression 1989 (updated)
Third impression 1989

British Library Cataloguing in Publication Data

Dowie, Robin
    Learning to live with multiple sclerosis.——
    Rev. ed.——(Overcoming common problems)
    1. Multiple sclerosis——Psychological aspects
    I. Title II. Povey, Robert   III. Prett,
    Gillian   IV. Dowie, Robin. Learning to live
    with MS   V. Series
    362.1'96834 RC377

    ISBN 0–85969–596–4

Typeset by Deltatype Limited, Ellesmere Port
Printed in Great Britain by
Richard Clay Ltd,
Bungay, Suffolk

Contents

Foreword

People with multiple sclerosis and their families are in great need of information, first of all about the strange disease that has entered their life and caused more or less profound changes. Just as important is the need to know how best to cope with the many problems of everyday life that inevitably arise. The authors of this book have wisely based their advice on answers provided by multiple sclerosis sufferers themselves and those who help them to maintain their independence. In this context practical wisdom is worth far more than medical knowledge. I have no doubt that those in need who read this book will derive much comfort and support.

Bryan Matthews
Professor of Clinical Neurology
University of Oxford

Acknowledgements

The inspiration for this book came from the members of the Canterbury and District Branch of the Multiple Sclerosis Society. Their warmth and spontaneity of friendship showed that multiple sclerosis was not to be feared but that the problems of living with it could be better understood. They gave their time and encouragement by preparing case histories about themselves and talking in groups about ways of coping with day-to-day tasks.

Marilyn Povey prepared the framework for the case histories. Then drawing on her personal experience as a sufferer and her professional knowledge as an occupational therapist she has offered ideas and advice at every stage in the preparation of the book. Valuable comments about the book were received from Dr Marion Hildick-Smith, Professor Michael Warren and Mrs Joan Warren, Professor Michael Drake and Mr John Walford. Secretarial assistance was given by Mrs Kathleen Horton and Mrs Joan Robson.

We are grateful for the help of all these people and for the encouragement of others who read the first draft of the book.

Canterbury, 1981

Preface to Second Edition

The first edition of this book was welcomed most enthusiastically by people with MS and their families, and about 3,000 copies have been sold in aid of the Canterbury and District branch of the MS Society. Since the publication of the original edition, however, some new and interesting areas of medical research have emerged. This second edition includes discussion of such developments (Chapter 2) and provides a revised up-to-date directory of benefits and allowances in Chapter 6. The remainder of the text has also been revised where necessary to take account of current developments in the management of MS.

We hope that the new edition will continue to prove helpful to MS sufferers and their families as well as to doctors, nurses, social workers, health visitors, physiotherapists, occupational therapists—in fact to anyone who cares for the disabled in a hospital or community setting.

1

The Doctor's Dilemma

Multiple sclerosis is a strange disorder. It doesn't have any really clear-cut symptoms in its early stages and it is very difficult to predict the likely course of the disease over a number of years. The problems experienced by one MS sufferer may be quite unlike those experienced by another. One person may show just a slow loss of mobility, gradually finding walking much more difficult, whereas another person might be confined to a wheel-chair for six months completely unable to walk and then be apparently fighting fit for another ten years or more. In these circumstances the doctor is faced with some difficult decisions. The guidelines for action are much less clear than they would be in the case of more straightforward ailments such as measles or mumps.

Diagnosis

The immediate problem confronting the doctor is that of making an accurate diagnosis. The first sign of MS may be something which can appear at times in healthy people such as an occasional numbness or feeling of pins and needles in the fingers or toes, or a slight and temporary disturbance of vision. Quite often such symptoms appear only fleetingly and it would be foolish for a doctor to jump to firm diagnostic conclusions on such flimsy evidence. Over a period of time, however, other symptoms may appear, often in different parts of the body, and these spasmodic episodes come to form a more coherent picture. It is then that one hopes that the general practitioner will play the 'detective' role and begin to piece together a few bits of the jigsaw. At this stage it is likely that the patient will be referred to the hospital consultant. In some cases, of course, the GP doesn't suspect the existence of MS at all. The symptoms being treated may appear, for example, as minor complications of quite common com-

1

plaints. Thus the tendency of MS patients to trip up over the corner of carpets or uneven pavements in the early stages of the disease may result in sprained ankles or broken bones which do not respond to treatment in the normal way. In such situations it may be the orthopaedic consultant at the hospital rather than the GP who suspects the existence of MS. The patient would then quite properly be referred to a more appropriate consultant—the neurologist.

Telling the patient

The diagnosis of neurological disease is an intricate and often time-consuming affair and even when the consultant has arrived at a diagnosis of MS the patient is sometimes not told that he or she has the disease. In some instances patients are sent away with their unexplained symptoms to contend with as a continuing source of anxiety. To the layman this seems a strange piece of behaviour by the medical profession but non-disclosure of the diagnosis to the patient used to be a very widespread practice. What then are the reasons for this particular approach?

In the first place the neurologist may not be completely certain about the diagnosis since the symptoms may be insufficiently clear. To tell a patient that he or she is suffering from a disabling disease when the neurologist is not quite certain about the diagnosis would obviously be wrong. Some form of follow-up examination is usually most appropriate in such circumstances. If, on the other hand, the neurologist is clear that the patient has MS then why should this diagnosis be concealed in such circumstances? The medical answer advanced by those neurologists who have supported the 'non-disclosure' approach seems to be that it is always possible that the symptoms which the patient is currently experiencing might disappear (in other words the patient might have a 'remission') and there may be a period of several months or years in which the patient is symptom-free. In these circumstances it would be better that the patient should not be worried unnecessarily about the possible long-term consequences of the disease. One MS sufferer, for example, had a ten-year remission in between the first symptoms appearing and their reappearance. The first symptoms of pins and needles, turning over an ankle and light-headedness lasted on and off for about a year and then apparently disappeared for the next ten! During those ten years she had a family, a part-time job, went cycling and dealt adequately with all the day-to-day chores of a housewife. Her own comment is: 'I'm glad I didn't know what exactly was wrong with me, as I might have kept worrying about when it would return.' This is the sort of case which provides some support for the medical practice of 'non-disclosure'.

However, many doctors and perhaps the majority of MS sufferers now believe that after a *firm* diagnosis has been made and the symptoms are becoming increasingly disabling then it is time for the doctor to take the patient into his or her confidence. Indeed there is evidence to suggest that failure to tell the patient can sometimes lead to distressing consequences. Thus one finds examples of MS sufferers finding out about their illness in a roundabout way: 'Doctors told me it was paraesthesia. This was over several years and many attacks. Multiple sclerosis was mentioned only when I applied for an invalid car . . . Finding it out only confirmed my suspicions. I resented being kept in the dark.' 'I was not told I had MS. I found out when I was rushed into hospital with peritonitis following an ectopic pregnancy. I overheard a nurse reading out my doctor's letter.'

Clearly, the discovery of MS by such roundabout routes is likely to be far more devastating in its effects than the discovery in the GP's surgery or the hospital clinic. Although it is difficult to generalise, the experience of MS sufferers does suggest that if the symptoms are well established 'being told' by the doctor can be a positive aid to the patient's adjustment. As one MS sufferer has said: 'It's my body and my life and I ought to have the right to know what's happening to them so that I can make an appropriate adjustment to the situation.' Indeed the person with MS often needs to have the aid of a diagnosis in order to make sense of the symptoms which still persist and cause anxiety despite the doctor's reassurance. Many MS sufferers in our survey drew attention to the sense of relief they have experienced at knowing what is wrong with them. They have been wondering whether they are suffering from brain tumours, cancer or mental illness. When they are told about MS the 'jigsaw pieces begin to fit together'. They can make sense of their symptoms and begin to adjust to their condition.

This adjustment is also something which can only be accomplished adequately if MS patients themselves are told about the disease. In the past the patient's relatives have sometimes been told without telling the patient but nowadays it is felt that this is usually an unnecessary burden to cast on the relatives. It increases anxiety without offering the possibility of constructive adjustment on the part of the whole family.

The doctor is certainly placed in a dilemma and there is no simple rule which can be applied in all cases. Doctors now believe, however, that in the past too many MS patients have been kept in the dark unnecessarily and given insufficient opportunity to come to terms with their disease.[1] Professor Bauer, for example, claims that it is important 'to provide the worried patients with more complete and truthful information . . . An evasive answer may cause many patients to worry even more, because they conclude that the doctor does not know what the disease is, or that his diagnosis implies such a bad prognosis, that the doctor does not dare to reveal the whole truth.' It is clear that sensitive judgement is required in relation to the treatment of patients as individuals. The doctor should, therefore, 'set aside time to convey to the patient and his family correct information about the disease and its consequences. The aim should be to encourage them not to lose their confidence and to give them a reasonable hope of being able to live with their disease.'

2

Some Information about the Disease

Once people have been told that they have multiple sclerosis, (disseminated sclerosis as it used to be called), then it is likely that they will be anxious to know more about the disease and why they should have got it. Unfortunately, multiple sclerosis is still not fully understood by medical doctors and scientists even though it was identified as a distinct disease by Charcot in Paris in 1868. This chapter provides a brief summary of what is known about the disease and those who suffer from it.[1] The chapter may seem rather technical but that is because the disease itself is complex.

Who are the sufferers?

In terms of the sex and age of newly diagnosed persons, most recent surveys agree that multiple sclerosis attacks women more frequently than men and on average at a slightly earlier age. For both sexes the risk of first developing symptoms rises steeply from early adolescence reaching a peak in the early thirties. The risk then falls away with increasing age.

MS sufferers and their families may feel anxious about whether the disease is inherited. There does not seem to be any direct inheritance because research on identical twins has shown that when one identical twin is affected the chance of the other twin having MS is little higher than in other brothers and sisters. However, MS does occur more often among the close relatives of those with the disease than in the general population and this may be due, in part, to exposure of the families to a common environmental influence. But it must be stressed that it is still very uncommon even among relatives.

Anyone who has dealings with multiple sclerosis sufferers quickly realises that the course and severity of the disease varies greatly between individuals. At one extreme it can cause severe

5

disabilities in a previously healthy adult; at the other extreme MS may have been present but undetected and the person may have lived to a ripe old age without suffering from any really disabling symptoms. In about one-tenth of cases the disorder is progressive from the start although with fluctuations, but the majority of sufferers have a history of relapses separated by stable periods (remissions) which can last for months or years. Indeed, some studies have shown that in about a quarter of cases the disease is benign and the sufferer has a normal life span with relatively little disability for ten or even twenty years or more after the initial appearance of the symptoms. In general, it seems that the degree of disability experienced five years after the first symptoms occur is a good index for the future. If a sufferer has only mild disability at five years then the disease is likely to remain mild although there will be exceptional cases.

Sufferers learn to cope with set-backs without necessarily going to see their family doctor. This is how one young woman described her health:

My remissions can last from anything up to two months to a year. Then I have a spasm which usually takes me in the leg, on occasions it has taken me in my right eye. Sometimes I can work these spasms off, other times I have to see the doctor and he gives me a few weeks off.

The general health record of many sufferers is about the same as that of people without MS. In our MS Branch, people who miss the occasional monthly meeting because of ill-health are nearly as likely to be able-bodied members as MS sufferers, and the reasons tend to be common ailments such as coughs and colds rather than the disease itself. It was shown in a survey of the work done by 115 general practitioners in 1970/1,[2] that patients with multiple sclerosis consulted their doctor about problems caused by the disease far less frequently than patients with other chronic disorders such as bronchitis, asthma, arthritis and Parkinson's disease (in the older age groups). But the reason for this may be that there is no truly satisfactory treatment for multiple sclerosis relapses.

Occasionally the newspapers or television carry stories about someone dying from multiple sclerosis, and these can give a misleading impression about the number of deaths caused by the disease. Only a tiny proportion of sufferers die from MS. It is much more likely for sufferers to die from common disorders such as respiratory or urinary infections, complications from fractures, and heart conditions.

What is multiple sclerosis?

The disease affects the nerves in the central nervous system, that is, in the brain and spinal cord. (It is not a mental disorder.) The nerves consist of bundles of microscopic nerve fibres and wrapping each fibre is a chemical sheath known as the myelin sheath. It is rather like the insulation protecting a telephone cable. The function of this myelin sheath is not fully understood but in MS some powerful agent attacks it, causing scarring with lesions or plaques being formed. As a result, many of the millions of fibres which run through the spinal cord fail to carry their messages clearly and various parts of the body cease to work properly.

It is thought that when somebody experiences his or her first symptoms, such as temporary loss of vision or a weakness in one or more limbs, there may be only one single plaque causing symptoms. When the symptoms recur especially if they are in a different part of the body, the doctors can be more certain that plaques have formed in more than one area; that is to say, they are multiple. There are sufferers, however, whose symptoms affect two or more parts of the body from the start. There is no specific test widely available to diagnose multiple sclerosis, a situation which applies to many disorders of the nervous system and to other illnesses. When diagnosing two or more lesion sites, doctors have had to depend on the way patients have described and demonstrated their symptoms. However, a technique has now been developed which measures the visually evoked responses of the brain as seen through the eye. This test can detect delayed responses caused by lesions or plaques in patients who are thought to be in the initial stages of multiple sclerosis. But the test is only available in specialised neurological centres and the results need to be interpreted in conjunction with the patients' accounts of their symptoms and the clinical evidence.

Even more recent has been the development of magnetic resonance imaging (MRI) which is a radiological imaging technique that detects the presence of hydrogen atoms in the body. The patient is placed in the field of a very powerful electro-magnet and subjected to short pulses of radio-frequency energy. When each pulse ends, the nuclei of the hydrogen atoms in the part of the body being examined send off signals and these are measured by a computer. In the brain, for example, grey matter contains more water than white matter and therefore more hydrogen. Using this technique, it is possible to identify lesions in the brain which were undetectable by other techniques. With MRI there is no risk of building up a dangerous dosage of radiation as there is with X-rays. So it can be used over and over again to assess patients' progress. Unfortunately, the cost of providing hospitals with MRI scanners is very high and there are very few hospitals in the United Kingdom equipped with one. But in 1983/4 the Multiple Sclerosis Society of Great Britain and Northern Ireland provided funds to install a scanner in the National Hospital for Nervous Diseases in London and the Society's commitment to MRI at the hospital now exceeds £2,000,000.

What causes multiple sclerosis?

Doctors and research scientists continue to be baffled about the cause of multiple sclerosis. The extensive research programmes throughout the world have not found out what causes the plaques to form nor why it happens in certain individuals. The search for answers has been held back because multiple sclerosis occurs exclusively in humans and so experiments on animals with the disease have not been possible although related animal diseases such as scrapie in sheep have been studied.

Studies of populations (epidemiological studies) suggest that there is an environmental factor. In terms of the world distribution of the disease, in the northern hemisphere, the British Isles and north and central Europe are in the high risk zone along with northern USA, Canada and Iceland and in the southern hemisphere, the high risk zone covers New Zealand and the Australian State of Tasmania. The disease is most common in white people. Studies have also shown that people who live in high risk areas in early life and then migrate to a low risk area still have a relatively high susceptibility to the disease.

It is estimated that in Great Britain about 100 persons in 100,000 suffer from MS. In the London Borough of Sutton a survey of the social services department, the local branch of the MS Society, general practitioners, hospital departments, community nurses and other sources gave an over-all prevalence figure of 115 per 100,000.[3] There are also small areas in the north with even higher rates of MS; for example, in the Orkney and Shetland Islands combined the figure is thought to be about 245 persons in 100,000, and for north-east Scotland over 120 per 100,000.

Other epidemiological evidence could suggest a genetic factor even though MS is not inherited. For instance, the overall risk of getting MS in Japan is very much lower than would be expected from the latitude of Japan. Furthermore, the Japanese still appear to have a low risk of developing the disease no matter where in the world they are born or live.

The population-based evidence has provided 'signposts' to valuable laboratory-based investigations. Just as everyone has a blood group so too we have tissue groups, and in the early 1970s it was discovered that MS occurs more frequently in one tissue group than in others. Then in 1975 work was started to identify the genes which determine tissue groups and six gene types were identified in the general population of south-east England. A remarkable finding was that over 80 per cent of patients with MS had one particular genetic factor as compared with about 33 per cent in the normal population. (This genetic factor is know as DRw2.)[4]

Anxious to validate these findings, the research team of

Professor W. I. McDonald, Professor D. A. S. Compston and Professor J. R. Batchelor went to Jordan to investigate an Arab population known to include MS sufferers. A genetic factor strongly associated with multiple sclerosis was established but the factor was different from the DRw2 factor which has now been found in all the groups of patients of northern European stock who have been examined except in the Orkneys and Shetlands where no association was found. In the Mediterranean, Italian MS sufferers have a genetic factor similar to that of the Jordanians but in Israeli patients there does not appear to be a consistent genetic factor. The genetic relationship in the few Japanese who have MS is different again. So it has been concluded that there are various genetic factors associated with MS and the association depends on the ethnic background of the patients. It is also acknowledged that there could be some other unidentified gene which is making the groups of people susceptible.

Another main line of research has been to find out if it is an environmental agent such as a virus that triggers the demyelination in the central nervous system causing the plaques to form. Since the mid 1960s teams of scientists have recovered from the brains of MS sufferers who had died at least nine different viruses or virus-like agents, including measles and herpes simplex. Unfortunately, no single virus-like body has been consistently isolated from MS brain specimens and shown to be different from objects seen in specimens of normal brain tissue. Nevertheless, much has been learnt about the interaction of viruses with cells in the brain.

There is now a theory that in some people (who may have similar genetic factors) a virus could be triggering the auto-immune responses that protect the body from infection and it is suggested that these responses themselves may cause the demyelination (the formation of the plaques).[5] This theory is supported by experimental work with a strain of a hepatitis virus that affects mice. It is possible to transfer immune cells from infected animals to healthy animals which then develop a chronic neurological disease resembling MS. This research, combined with other experiments on viral agents affecting small animals, serves as a model for studying MS. Much more work has yet to be done in this field but if a specific viral agent was identified, then it might be possible to develop a vaccine against MS just as the measles and poliomyelitis vaccines were produced.

Treatment in MS

The other major research area has been concerned with learning about the process of demyelination so that a treatment can be developed which will stop the process or, better still, reverse it. An effective treatment for multiple sclerosis could possibly be developed before the cause of the disease has been established. So far, research has failed to show conclusively how the myelin breaks down and the plaques form, with the result that any treatments which have been tried have only been experimental. An Australian team conducted a two-year trial in which a group of MS patients were given injections of a white cell (leucocyte) extract obtained from relatives living with them. Another group of patients received placebo injections (blank injections) and neither group knew whether it was receiving the extract or the placebo injections. The 'transfer factor' in the extract appeared to gradually slow down the progression of the disease in patients with mild to moderate disability but relapses continued to occur in the treated group.

One line of treatment has been diet. The myelin sheath is made up mostly of fatty material including polyunsaturated fats and in regions of the world where the diet of the population as a whole is very low in saturated fatty acids, the disease is relatively rare. As a consequence there have been various trials of unsaturated fats, notably sunflower seed oil containing linoleic acid, and Naudicelle capsules containing oil from the evening primrose. Gluten-free diets have also been tried.

Although many persons have felt better while taking these dietary agents and there is no evidence to show that the diets caused any harm, there is still a lack of conclusive scientific evidence that the diets actually interrupted the disease process within their bodies. Unfortunately, this evidence will be difficult to obtain because of the erratic nature of the disease itself. As the pattern of relapses and remissions in any one person cannot be predicted, there is no way of knowing whether diet has actually held back the disease or a natural remission period has been reached. However, as some researchers are so convinced that diet may be one way forward, a project was set up in 1980 in the Central Middlesex Hospital, London, by the charity ARMS (Action for Research into Multiple Sclerosis). The aim of the project was to study the relationship between diet and multiple sclerosis, and the progress of MS patients has been monitored after they have received nutritional advice including a suggested change from saturated to polyunsaturated fats and a reduction of foods containing sugar. The main finding from this research was that people who followed the dietary advice well remained neurologically stable over the three years of the study, while those who didn't experienced a decline in their neurological state.

The same problem of measuring the effects occurs when steroid drug treatments are given to patients who are having a relapse. These steroid drugs act upon the immunological processes and they include cortisone-based preparations such as prednisolone and prednisone, and a pituitary gland preparation known as ACTH. One reason why it is difficult to judge the benefits of these drugs is that they are not usually given to a patient until a relapse has begun, so there is no way of knowing if the recovery was the result of the drug or just the natural course of the disease.

There have been medical trials in which a group of MS sufferers were given a steroid preparation over a year or more. In one trial the anti-viral agent known as interferon was administered to patients in weekly lumbar puncture injections. Many of these trials have not included a *control* group of sufferers (that is, persons not receiving the treatment). This has meant that the relapse rates of two groups of treated and untreated patients could not be compared. The interferon trial did have a control group who received placebo lumbar puncture injections, and the patients who had the active treatment had many fewer relapses in the follow-up period. But the number of patients involved was very small—ten in each group—and so the trial can only be considered to have been a pilot trial. Another difficulty about the results of medical trials is that groups of MS patients in general tend to experience fewer relapses as time goes by.

However, very many MS sufferers have received courses of ACTH or the other steroid preparations, during the period of a relapse from their neurologist or general practitioner, with seemingly encouraging benefits. Injections of vitamin B_{12} too, are often prescribed during relapses as this vitamin has been found to be important in the recovery of the spinal cord from other causes of degeneration. But for the majority of different kinds of symptoms that might trouble MS sufferers, the treatments are the same as those given to persons with other diseases: for example, antibiotics for urinary infections; Cetiprin or ephedrine derivatives for minor urinary incontinence; and tranquillisers or anti-depressants for severe emotional difficulties. Experiments were carried out to stimulate the dorsal area of the spinal cord by electrodes and there was evidence to suggest that the treatment improved, at least temporarily, some body functions including the bladder in the more severely disabled. However, the results overall were disappointing and there are risks of infection associated with the treatment.

In the late 1970s considerable interest was roused in the use of hyperbaric oxygen to treat MS sufferers. It was thought that since oxygen breathed at twice the atmospheric pressure (that is, hyperbaric oxygen) produces a high concentration of oxygen in the body, it would delay the demyelination process. One theory behind the treatment was that the MS plaques result from a blocking of blood vessels, causing a lack of oxygen. By the early 1980s treatment was being provided in centres across the country. The commonly used method was to fill a pressure chamber similar to those used in deep sea diving, with air under pressure and for the sufferers to breathe oxygen through a mask while in the chamber. The usual course of treatment was 90 minutes per day for five days a week for a total of six weeks.

Since there are risks associated with the decompression treatment especially for MS patients who suffer from chronic ear or sinus disease, asthma, chronic bronchitis or emphysema, it was considered important that the treatment should be scientifically evaluated. So various trials were set up in Britain and overseas. The MS Society assisted with the funding of at least two trials involving control groups in hospitals in London. At the beginning of 1986 a paper was published reporting the results of one of these trials in which an experimental group breathed oxygen while in a pressurised chamber and the placebo group breathed normal air also while in the pressurised chamber but at a different time. Each group received twenty treatment sessions over a four-week period. The results were disappointing. No significant improvements were found in the patients who had received the oxygen although a few had a slightly increased bladder capacity. Both groups of patients experienced unwanted effects from the treatment. Minor ear discomfort and fatigue were the commonest problems.[6] Thus the results from this trial and from other trials in the United Kingdom, Sweden and the USA unfortunately do not support the claims made for hyperbaric oxygen in the management of MS.

Despite the fact that no major research breakthrough has been achieved, it is encouraging to note that very considerable progress has been made in the past decade in understanding viral diseases, the immunological processes in the body, and the pathology of the central nervous system—all of which have a direct relevance to multiple sclerosis. In the meantime, until the mystery of MS begins to unravel more fully, physiotherapy remains the cornerstone of treatment—helping the patients to make the most of the strengths that they have. Attention to one's general diet is also recommended.

The breakthrough in the medical treatment of many common diseases (such as gout and stomach ulcers) tends to come, of course, from a 'brick-by-brick laying' process of new information over a number of years by scientists in various specialised fields. For multiple sclerosis this pattern of joint research is now in progress. The two major funding bodies in this country are the

Multiple Sclerosis Society of Great Britain and Northern Ireland and the government's Medical Research Council. During each of the three years 1982–4 the MS Society allocated just over £1,000,000 to research and by 1988 this figure had risen to around £3,000,000 per year. In addition there is international co-operation through both the scientific journals and conferences, and the International Federation of Multiple Sclerosis Societies. So there is every reason to hope for a breakthrough in the not-too-distant future.

3

MS and the Family

MS sometimes strikes before thoughts of marriage or starting a family have become important. More usually, however, it appears at a time when two people may be contemplating marriage or a husband and wife are considering how to plan the family. For the couple about to get married the burning issue is what effect MS is likely to have on their married life.

MS and marriage

As mentioned in the previous chapter MS is neither an infectious nor a contagious disease and there is therefore no danger of the transmission of the disease from one partner to the other. It is a disease, however, which makes great demands upon sufferers and their close family and friends. Some people find disability of any sort difficult to contend with and may shrink away from the prospect of painful, emotional or physical experiences. In general, MS is not a disorder which inflicts unbearable pain although nagging pain of a toothache kind is not uncommon. It does, on the other hand, present considerable problems of adjustment on social, financial, sexual and emotional matters. Such adjustments are generally much easier to make in the context of a loving and supportive relationship as, for example, in a good marriage. If the bond between two people is sufficiently strong and based upon values and interests which are not just transitory then marriage with MS can be a great success despite the difficulties. If the bonds between two individuals are flimsy, however, and based upon little more than physical attraction the chances of maintaining a steady relationship in the midst of MS are much less good. The decision about whether to marry or not must be an individual decision based upon careful consideration of the circumstances. To write off marriage simply because one partner has this disease would be a very shallow way of looking at

16

the problem and there are many instances of highly successful and fulfilled marriages or relationships in which one partner has MS.

The first problem which will face a couple is how to accept the initial diagnosis. This can often be a devastating experience. Sometimes the information is acquired when the patient is least ready to accept it (for example when suffering from a sudden relapse or when in hospital for another apparently unconnected complaint). It would be helpful if some form of counselling service were available at such times but constructive advice tends to be very limited. Some GPs are very good and some nurses or social workers can be helpful at such a time of stress. The local branch of the MS Society can also be of great assistance and the opportunity to talk with another MS sufferer can be a considerable help.

The first thing to accept, of course, is that it is quite natural to feel depressed and even rather desperate on first hearing about MS. On examining the possible consequences of the disease, however, it usually becomes clear that the picture which is sometimes painted of rapid and drastic deterioration in the condition is less than accurate in most cases.

The very worst thing to do would be to look in an out-of-date medical dictionary at this time! Before you know where you are you will be condemned to a wheelchair as a prelude to becoming permanently bedridden in no time at all. Fortunately the majority of MS cases are much less dramatic! There may be very little disability in the early stages. Difficulty in walking and perhaps some urgency in needing to go to the toilet may be the main problems at such a stage and in some cases a remission can mean that the person does not even suffer these limitations. People often find it helpful to talk about their anxieties openly to their partner or to an understanding doctor, social worker or MS society member. Many of the worst fears are unfounded and it is important to try to obtain a reliable picture of the sort of problems with which the MS sufferer has to cope. It is also important to realise that the period of adjustment to the initial medical diagnosis of MS will differ in length according to the

17

individual concerned. For most people it seems to take about two years before it is possible to talk easily to relatives and friends about the illness. The feelings of fear, anger and inadequacy which are often very strong at first wear off in time and it becomes easier and easier to discuss the problems of MS with other people. The illness can then become a challenge to which many people both inside and outside the family will respond most strongly, and don't forget that in many cases the symptoms subside for long periods (sometimes permanently) and in others they will remain fairly static. So the story is often less gloomy than it might at first appear.

The role of the partner in MS

There is sometimes an understandable tendency for the partner of an MS sufferer to 'molly-coddle the invalid'. In many cases this has the unfortunate effect of reducing the degree of independence of the person with MS who becomes labelled as a 'patient' incapable of carrying out normal household or occupational activities. This can lower the morale of the person and in certain ways lead to a deterioration in his or her physical condition. In fighting this illness it is extremely important that the MS sufferer should keep as fully involved in the activities formerly engaged in for as long as possible. For example, cooking or cleaning might take a great deal longer than it used to but the exercise that such activities provide for mind and muscles is extremely important in the maintenance of physical and mental well-being. Watching the person with MS doing jobs at an excruciatingly slow pace can be most frustrating for the onlooker as well as the individual. Too frequently this leads the onlooker to exclaim 'let me do it' and to take over the task which is consequently accomplished much more swiftly. It is phrases and actions such as these which require curbing on the part of the able-bodied partner. Nothing can dent the morale of an MS sufferer more than the gradual loss of responsibilities. Rather than take over the task it is often more constructive to try to find ways of making that task easier (for example, by using an electric mixer instead of a wooden spoon).

In general it is true, however, that for every disabled person it is helpful if there is someone around who is able-bodied. One of the adjustments which the MS sufferer has to make is to learn to accept help when it is needed. This is often a most difficult adjustment to make. Many people with MS become fiercely independent and sometimes seem to reject offers of help in a startlingly brusque manner. To those who live with MS this might be accepted simply as an assertion of independence; to those unconnected with MS it appears to be rudeness. The person with MS needs to come to terms with the fact that help is sometimes required and to accept it gracefully.

In the situation where the role of husband and wife can often be virtually reversed it is not surprising that tensions will creep into the relationship. Such tensions are perfectly natural. People with MS often tend to feel guilty about the extra burden which is being placed on their partner. On the other hand, the able-bodied partner may sometimes feel annoyed and resentful at having to forgo leisure activities because of family commitments. The husband or wife can sometimes also be over-sensitive to criticism. A husband may feel, for example, that he is doing enough simply to take on some extra household chores without being criticised for doing them in a manner which is at variance with his wife's usual approach. People with MS in these circumstances have to accept that tasks which they have per-formed earlier on in the marriage and to their own particular standards will now be performed by their spouse in *their* own way. It is often small points like the way in which clothes are hung out on the line or how the car is cleaned which will present the most irritating points of conflict. Pride has often to be swallowed and critical tongues bitten in order to cope with such tensions. Given understanding and good humour, however, they need not become permanent complications.

MS does not respect privacy in a marriage. One of the things which husbands and wives might have to accept is that MS may necessitate the assistance of the partner with some of the body's basic functions. Difficulty in reaching the toilet on time can be a problem in MS and coupled with the difficulty in physical movement of arms and legs this may make assistance with clothing necessary. Bathing, getting in and out of bed, sometimes eating and drinking—all these may require assistance to a greater or lesser degree. 'And one man in his time plays many parts.' *(As You Like It,* Act II, scene 7.)

Sexual relations between partners need not necessarily be affected by MS. The functioning of the body in this respect may remain perfectly normal although there may be difficulties in some cases. Occasionally male sufferers may find impotence occurs. This is not, of course, only a problem for MS sufferers and it is something which may be amenable to treatment. Even if it is not possible to treat this problem the possibility of engaging in satisfactory sexual relations is not something to discard. The GP can be of help in these matters and there are some useful pamphlets which give advice to the disabled in sexual matters (for example, *Forum,* 1975; SPOD).[1]

One of the main problems in sexual matters is physical discomfort and fatigue. The claim that 'I'm too tired tonight' is something which tends to have rather more justification in MS than might always be the case in other situations! As in all aspects of the relationship, therefore, adjustments have to be made to this area of activity.

A final point on the relationship between partners concerns the fact that many MS sufferers are unable to leave the house on their own. In these circumstances the able-bodied partner often acts as the eyes and ears of the person with MS. It is important to spend time discussing things which are taking place in the local town or village so that the MS sufferer feels involved in the outside world. Visits to places of interest or even a drive around the houses with no particular destination in mind can be like a trip to Buckingham Palace to see the Queen for somebody who is generally housebound. It is important also to try to overcome the embarrassment husbands or wives may feel when taking their partners to social occasions. MS sufferers have the problem of coming to terms with their own self-image as disabled and their partners have the parallel problem of adjusting to the disability and to other people's reactions to it. In order to come to terms with this problem it is sometimes necessary to force oneself into accepting invitations despite the initial reservations. As time progresses and the circle of understanding acquaintances increases social activities become easier to cope with. At this stage fatigue is more a problem than embarrassment.

Children and MS

The question about whether or not to have children is one which some people with MS have to face. Medical opinion in general gives no strong guidance either way. Adoption agencies, on the other hand, tend to reject parents with MS on the grounds that they have enough able-bodied applicants to provide their children with adoptive parents. As far as pregnancy is concerned in a woman with MS, medical advice needs to be sought with respect to each individual case. Sometimes pregnancy may be inadvisable; on the other hand there are many cases in which pregnancy and childbirth appear to have little or no effect on the course of the disease. It is the period following the child's birth which creates the greatest problem for the mother with MS. For a mother in good health this period is very fatiguing; for the mother with MS it becomes even more fatiguing and the family need to rally round at this time to give as much assistance as possible.

The other general consideration the prospective parents have to bear in mind is whether it is right to bring a child into the world into circumstances where the couple may find it difficult to cope with the upbringing of children because of the disability or where the family may be at risk financially because of the parent's illness. Each case needs to be considered on its own merit. However, any disadvantages to the child's upbringing which may result from the physical frailty of a parent or from financial hardship will be more than off-set in the long term by the security and emotional warmth provided by a loving family.

In making a decision about whether or not to have children it is wise to take into account the long-term as well as the short-term future, to make sure that the decision is a joint one and that there are people within the family who would help out in times of difficulty. Family planning also becomes very important in the case of families where one of the members has MS. This is another reason why it is important for sufferers to be told they have MS as soon as the symptoms are well established and a firm diagnosis has been made.

In general the children of MS families seem to develop healthily and happily. As we have already noted, MS is not inherited and the disease is not passed on from mother to child. There are, however, certain aspects of growing up which such children might miss out on. For example it is not as easy for a parent with MS to take the children out or to visit school functions as an able-bodied parent. Children have to learn to be independent at an early age and this can often be a great aid to the development of maturity. It can also sometimes lead to a feeling that they are being imposed upon. The danger of placing too much responsibility on the children is something of which MS parents (mothers in particular) are often acutely aware. The parents may also sometimes feel rather guilty that they are not able to do everything they would like for their children because of the limitations imposed by the disability.

There is, however, a very *positive* side to bringing up children in a family where one parent has MS. Living with disability seems to give children a sensitivity to the needs of other people which is less easily acquired in able-bodied families. If children have known their parents as MS sufferers from their early childhood then it is likely that they will accept the disability and its consequences without too much frustration or embarrassment.

Children can often be disconcertingly frank. Whereas adults will refrain from remarking upon abnormalities of physique or gait for fear of embarrassing, the inquisitive child will simply ask in a straightforward way 'why do you walk like that?' or 'why have you got a stick?' Such curiosity is best answered by straightforward explanations: 'I've got a funny leg', 'My legs won't work properly'. As the children get older more precise information about MS can be discussed and children show a good understanding of the problems involved and will often spend time thinking how to cope with them. For example, one little boy friendly with a family in which the mother has MS always looked to see if the places he visited on school and family outings were accessible for a wheelchair. The daughter of an MS mother exclaimed 'When I grow up I'm going to buy a house without any steps so that mummy will be able to come and visit me'. Wheelchairs are constant sources of interest to children. Unlike many adults who seem to shun people in wheelchairs out of embarrassment children seem drawn towards them out of wonder and curiosity at this interesting form of transport.

Although some children of MS parents may show anxiety about their parent's condition to an excessive degree most seem to accept the position in a fairly well balanced way. They will have their periods of anxiety about what would happen if there was a fire, whether mummy will have to go into hospital, what happens if daddy dies—but this is not greatly different from the fears and worries of children in ordinary households. The drawbacks which children suffer from having a parent who is more housebound than most other parents are counterbalanced by advantages such as the certainty that this parent will always be at home when the child comes home from school! In general the development of independence, responsibility and sensitivity to the needs of others seem great bonuses to set against the minor frustrations.

The role of relatives and friends

The parents of MS sufferers often seem to feel as much of a shock as the patients themselves at the time of the initial diagnosis. It is also the experience of MS sufferers that parents are often among the most difficult with whom to discuss the illness because of their emotional involvement. They sometimes seem not to want to talk about the disease and to pretend that it is not there. Another reaction is to want to take the person back in to the parental home so that they can look after them 'properly'. This overprotective urge is something which parents need to guard against. Although the task of looking after a daughter or son with

MS may fulfil a parental need it can also reduce the independence of the individual MS sufferer. For the parent pushing their daughter or son around in a wheelchair may seem a helpful and unselfish gesture but to the person in the wheelchair it may seem too closely related to childhood experiences to be seen in this way. The person with MS will usually appreciate the 'unfussy' approach much more than the 'cottonwool treatment' even though this may seem slightly harsh to the parents. This is how one MS sufferer puts it:

> The most important attitude of all . . . in dealing with those of us who are handicapped, is that which treats us as far as possible as if we enjoyed normal health . . . It is certainly my experience that we who are handicapped are happier and healthier if, up to a point, we are 'treated rough', and not only encouraged but *expected* to do things for ourselves, without any fuss or comment being made about what we do.

Relatives generally can be a tremendous source of support to the family with MS if they try to understand the particular problems of MS such as fatigue. They can often provide a very effective back up service to the immediate family stepping in as 'babysitters' or 'food suppliers' or 'transporters' at times of difficulty. Close friends can also be tremendously helpful. It's not the person who goes on her 'do-gooding' visit with a bunch of flowers who is of most value to the MS sufferer but the friend who says 'I'm just going shopping—is there anything I can get you?' The flower person fatigues, the shopper prevents fatigue. The real friend is one who is willing to come in and mop up the dog's puddle because the person with MS can't get down to do this. It is helpful also for friends to remember that sitting chatting over a cup of tea for a couple of hours can be extremely tiring for some people with MS. Another important point is that the ordinary colds and 'flus which most people take in their stride may be more of a problem for the person with MS. A bout of 'flu can be very debilitating for an MS sufferer and it is, therefore, important that people should not bring such germs into the household where someone has MS.

It is quite common for people to find that they lose one or two friends after MS has been diagnosed. Some probably are unable to face up to any discussion of illness and keep away out of fear and embarrassment. Other friends seem to be insufficiently aware of the nature of the disease. The main problem of MS, according to one sufferer, is 'trying to explain to other people why I can't do the things I used to'!

Although MS clearly has very considerable effects on family life it is important to stress that there are very many families coping successfully with the problems and some families have come closer together as a consequence of them.

4

Coping and Hoping

In MS one has to cope with the immediate consequences of the disease whilst at the same time keeping alive the hope that research will come up with the cause and some pointers to treatment. It is therefore very much a position of coping and hoping.

General problems

As far as coping is concerned this depends very much upon the nature of the symptoms in each particular case. It depends also upon the home, occupational circumstances and the stage of the illness. For example, the requirements for coping with someone in a wheelchair are rather different from those in which the person is able to walk short distances. The symptoms are many and varied but there are one or two features which seem common to most people with MS—fatigue, poor balance and difficulty in walking, for example, are basic problems. MS sufferers sometimes have difficulty in locating their limbs in relation to the rest of their body; pins and needles and heaviness of the limbs are also a common occurrence. These symptoms lead to many instances of dropped crockery, headlong falls after tripping over carpets or down pavements. Fingers sometimes lack sensation and may become progressively weaker in grasping objects and in close coordination. This can lead to difficulty in dressing, performing ordinary household tasks such as cutting bread, sewing, hairwashing. Circulation is often poor and this can lead to excessively cold or excessively hot feet and hands and some swelling of the limbs.

Many MS sufferers are also adversely affected by hot sun. Sometimes vision may be impaired (by temporary bouts of double vision) and this can affect leisure pursuits such as reading or watching television. People with MS can also have problems with cramps, 'floppy' limbs or stiffness of the muscles. Stiffness is a very common problem which can affect mobility in many ways. For example, in the morning some MS sufferers find that their legs are as stiff as planks at first, and before they can get up from bed they will need assistance in bending their legs. Physical discomfort can also affect sleeping at night. Frequency and urgency in going to the toilet are also common and very difficult problems as is the general overriding problem of fatigue.

Another problem, especially in the early stages of MS, is that many of the symptoms such as fatigue and weakness in bladder control are invisible to other people.

> The presence of these invisible symptoms may cause anxiety, and the patient may not know whether to perceive himself as 'disabled' or 'fit'. He may alternate between the two roles depending on domestic and work circumstances. Sometimes he fails to make allowances for the disease . . . by working too hard or by engaging in stressful activities to prove that he is 'normal'. He may think that if he mentions his tiredness or subjective symptoms he will be regarded as a hypochondriac or as a malingerer.[1]

This description may be representative of the state of mind of some MS sufferers early on in the course of the disease. But over a period of time people with MS, their families, workmates and friends gradually come to terms with the symptoms, both visible and invisible, and many of the conflicts tend to resolve themselves.

With such a range of symptoms, however, it is difficult to give general guidance about coping strategies and this chapter will take different aspects of everyday life in turn and try to offer certain hints which might be of help to people with MS. There are, however, one or two general comments which might be of help. Perhaps the most important practical step that can be taken is to try to make the physical side of life as convenient as possible. Since lack of mobility and a tendency to become overtired are central features in the illness it is common sense to try to equip the home with as many labour-saving devices as possible. Another general point is the need to avoid over-tiredness. This means planning one's day well in advance and as carefully as possible so that periods of work can be interspersed with periods of rest throughout the day. If MS is regarded as a challenge and tackled positively and constructively it is usually possible to find ways of coping with even the most difficult problems.

Physical health and diet

Since the physical health of MS sufferers is already impaired by the disease it is crucial to try to keep the general level of health as high as possible. In this respect it is helpful to lead a life with as few extra stresses as possible and with as much activity as is compatible with the avoidance of over fatigue. Physiotherapy is often recommended for MS patients and it seems sensible to try to keep the muscles in trim so that they are ready for action in the event of remission. The problem with physiotherapy is that it must not overtire the patient and frequently physiotherapy requires visiting a hospital quite a long way from home. In some cases the energy required for this journey tends to defeat the object of the exercise. Some MS sufferers find that swimming or hydrotherapy is a help and others use exercise machines in their own homes. Yoga is something else which has been found helpful by a number of people with MS.[2] Certain vitamin supplements are recommended in MS. Most of these will be found in chemists under names such as 'Multivite'. One vitamin supplement which may be of special value in MS is vitamin B_{12} and this can be taken orally or by injection. The doctor will also sometimes prescribe ACTH injections for MS patients and in cases of relapse this can be beneficial.

Research has shown the value of certain dietary approaches in MS and it has been established that sunflower seed oil can be marginally helpful to MS sufferers in certain circumstances. Since this is available commercially as oil in margarine and can be used in cooking this is obviously a sensible dietary supplement. The gluten-free diet has not received medical support as treatment for MS although several sufferers use the diet and claim that it is beneficial in their cases. The person with MS should aim generally to eat a healthy diet, keeping it low in animal fats, for example, and including plenty of white fish and green vegetables. Food high in natural fibre, such as bran and wholemeal bread, can also be useful in preventing constipation, and it is important to control the diet so that the person's weight is kept fairly constant. Excessive weight can increase the sufferer's difficulties in walking and create added problems for the helper who is trying to assist in lifting or moving the person with MS.

Occupation

Most people with MS would probably say that it is important to keep involved with a job for as long as possible. It depends, of course, upon the type of job and the severity of the MS symptoms. One MS sufferer, for example, managed to conceal his difficulties in walking for some time but eventually his drunken gait was too pronounced for him to remain as a police officer on patrol duty! In this case and in many similar cases people with MS have been fortunate in transferring to lighter duties within the same occupational setting. The advice from one person with MS to somebody in their late twenties or early thirties who had just discovered they had MS was that they should 'Think ahead. You probably won't get a lot worse, but you might do, so if there's a possibility that you'll not be as good as you are now, then try and look ahead and train yourself or get yourself trained for something you can do even then, when you are not as agile as you are now.'[3] Planning ahead is clearly a key factor in the selection of an occupation. Physically tiring occupations and those involving finely coordinated movements are likely to be found difficult but many occupations (for example, desk jobs and telephone operating tasks) may be quite applicable. One MS sufferer, indeed, ran a business from his home with the aid of a possum machine.

Housework

The main guideline here is to invest in labour-saving devices. For most people freezers, automatic washing machines and tumble driers would be regarded as luxuries. For the person with MS these take on the mantle of necessities. Unfortunately they are expensive necessities and many people with MS are unable to afford them. This is where some of the local charities, including the MS Society, can sometimes help. The local authority social services may also be able to assist with some home conversions or gadgets. One very difficult problem for MS sufferers, for example, is the retrieval of objects from the floor. If they try to bend down to pick them up they inevitably land up on the floor themselves and are unable then to haul themselves back into the chair! One gadget which the local authority can supply is a pick-up stick which has a long handle and acts like pincers. The local authority can also supply certain walking aids to provide stability for the MS sufferer. Where available the Community Occupational Therapist will be able to give advice on this.

Making beds is another problem for people with MS. They are often unable to bend down to the level of the bed without toppling over and if one hand is weak then tucking in bedclothes becomes an impossibility. One answer here is to invest in continental quilts. Hanging out clothes on the washing line is another problem for some people with MS. A tumble drier will remove the necessity for this activity if finances and space permit. A helpful neighbour is another possibility. For someone who can just manage to reach the washing line it might be easier to put the clothes pegs on the clothes before approaching the line. Putting the clothes on a trolley and wheeling this to the clothes line is also something which many people have found helpful. Indeed, trollies are transports of magnificent worth for anyone suffering from MS. They provide a ready-built walking frame, a conveyor of food and drink, and a most effective extension of the hands and arms when carrying clothes, plants, books from one part of the house to another.

When it comes to ironing the answer is to sit down at the ironing board—a procedure which seems to leave many stand-up traditionalists aghast! The other solution to ironing is to buy clothes which in general are of the 'non-iron' variety—poly-cotton sheets, drip-dry shirts and so on. If you have the

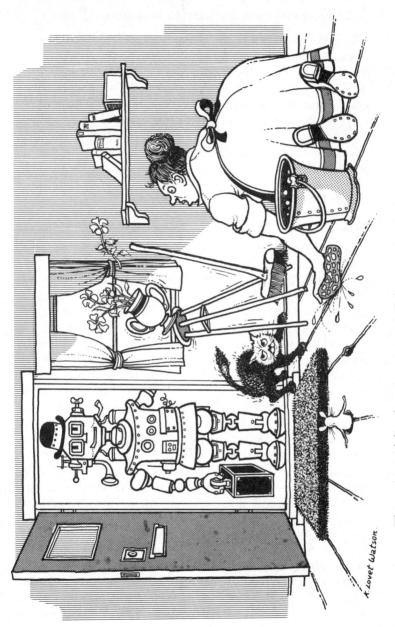

The main guideline here is to invest in labour-saving devices.

K. Lovet Watson.

opportunity to decide where electric sockets are placed then it is helpful to raise these a couple of feet or so off the ground so that they are more accessible to a disabled person. For example, if the person is in a wheelchair then he or she would still be able to plug in a vacuum cleaner and push it in front of the wheelchair.

Another aid to housework is the home help and a great many people with MS have found the local authority service helpful in this respect. One MS sufferer describes her home help as 'an absolute necessity and ministering angel'. The home help can provide a regular social contact for many people as well as a housework, shopping and cooking aid.

Cooking

The weakness in the hands of many MS sufferers can cause problems with carrying pans and mixing ingredients whilst the problems of fatigue can cause difficulties in preparing regular meals. Everything takes three or four times as long in MS as in an able-bodied context and this also adds to the problems of fatigue. Thus the use of electrical gadgets is clearly of great assistance in the kitchen (and if finance is a problem don't forget that you can ask for help from organisations such as your local MS branch). The difficult-to-operate tin-opener can be replaced by an electric tin-opener, the wooden spoon and bowl can be replaced by an electric mixer, the fridge can be supplemented by a freezer, the oven by a microwave. For working on kitchen surfaces it is often helpful to sit on a high stool since standing at the sink or kitchen table can soon result in exhaustion. If finances can allow the purchase of a freezer then it is possible to cut down one's work fairly dramatically by preparing several meals at the same time and freezing them. For example, if a casserole or bolognese is being prepared then enough can be cooked for three or four meals. The effort involved in preparing this amount is very little different from that involved in preparing for one meal yet the result will be the production of two or three extra meals for future occasions. The same will apply to cake mixtures and many other foods. Even sandwiches can be frozen in bulk for use at a later date. In this way special occasions such as Christmas and birthdays can be planned well in advance and much of the last minute work and effort can be removed.

Peeling vegetables is something which people with MS may find difficult. One solution is to resort to baked potatoes rather than peeled and to sample the wide variety of frozen or tinned vegetables on the market. Packs of oven-baked or frozen chips can also save a great deal of effort. The danger with fat-fried chips is that a pan full of hot fat can be a dangerous hazard in the kitchen. One person with MS fell and struck her head whilst frying chips and lay concussed with a pan of sizzling fat just above her head. She remained there until her husband came home at lunchtime. The moral of this tale seems to be—don't fry chips unless accompanied or get a member of the family to bring them home from the fish and chip shop! One or two kitchen tips are to cook the vegetables in a chip basket placed in a saucepan of water or use a strainer spoon to take the vegetables from the pan instead of trying to tip out the water first; to put a mixing bowl on a rubber sticking mat or in the sink when mixing; to make custard like porridge by mixing the powder with the milk in the pan and heating them up together rather than mixing the custard in a jug and then pouring on the hot milk. A final hint on cooking from a woman with MS: 'the milkman is quite good in the kitchen . . . he opens tins . . . he gets things out of the deep freeze . . . he zips me up the back'!

Living accommodation

Few people are given the opportunity to design their own homes and fewer still have the opportunity to do so with the knowledge that MS has arrived or is lurking nearby. Most people, therefore, have to make do with the accommodation they have and with various modifications to this. The local authority Social Services Department may well be able to help with these modifications. Detailed information about such local authority assistance is given in Chapter 6 together with other information relevant to living accommodation and the disabled (for example, the availability of rate rebates). If it is possible to influence decisions about the type of living accommodation to be obtained,

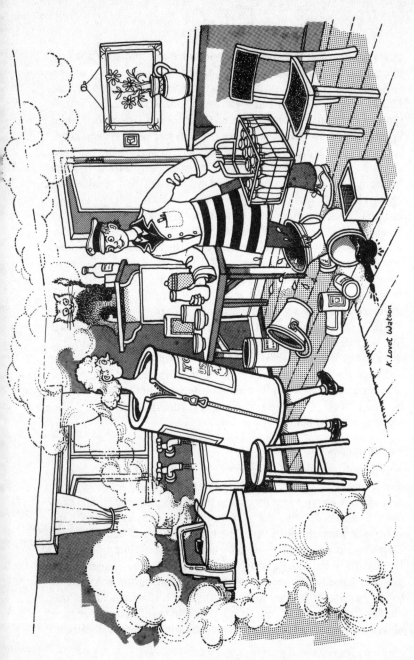

K. Lovet Watson

. . . he zips me up the back!

however, then there are certain points which if would be helpful to bear in mind. Since difficulty in walking is one of the main problems of MS then facilities downstairs and on the level are a priority. At some point the majority of MS sufferers find stairs difficult to negotiate. If the bedroom is upstairs and the only toilet is upstairs then two of the most important rooms in the house are virtually inaccessible. Chairlifts are now being supplied with the aid of some local authorities and these can ease the problems. Similarly it may be possible to build in a downstairs toilet by converting a stair cupboard or building a porch extension which incorporates a cloakroom and toilet. Local authorities are often willing to assist with such conversions for the disabled. If there is a choice about whether to have a shower installed as a washing facility then advantage should be taken of this since the use of a bath becomes increasingly difficult for many MS sufferers.

Frequently a bungalow offers an ideal solution and this would be particularly important with the advent of a wheelchair. Wheelchair use also requires a reasonable width in door space although nowadays with 'slim-line' chairs a normal width of doorway is sufficient. Entrance into the house and garage needs to be as level as possible and even if not required for wheelchair use level entrances are generally most convenient. Steps are the constant nightmare of people with MS as with other physically handicapped people and the elderly. Slippery floors and rugs are also a danger to the MS sufferer and these are to be avoided.

Kitchen design is something which could be vastly improved in many instances to the benefit of the disabled (and able-bodied) person. Since heavy pans cannot be handled easily it is important that the person with MS should be able to slide the pans from one part of the kitchen to another along a working surface. A useful arrangement is one planned in the following sequence: cooker—surface—sink —surface—fridge. An oven design which many people have found helpful is one in which the oven door flap comes down so that it is possible to rest casserole dishes on this.

The phone is also essential. This provides a contact with the outside world and a reassurance of help in times of distress. One problem about the telephone is that the person with MS is often unable to reach the telephone before the caller has rung off. When walking is very impaired this can be a most frustrating experience. The use of a 'cordless' portable telephone is one answer. Another is the careful placement of telephones. For example, a telephone might be placed in the kitchen and the telephone engineers asked to leave a long extension cable so that the telephone can be transported from the kitchen to the lounge by using a trolley. It is possible also to provide extra sockets in other rooms such as the bedroom so the telephone can be moved. It is still worth reminding friends of MS sufferers that they need to keep on ringing to allow the person to reach the phone. The emergency use of the phone can be reduced in effectiveness, of course, if the person trips before reaching the phone. In such circumstances it is useful if the children are well drilled in the '999' call procedure. It has also been found helpful to wear a whistle round the neck so that the attention of a neighbour can be attracted in a way other than by using the phone. More sophisticated electronic devices such as the AID-call system[4] may be offered to disabled people by some Local Authorities.

Toilet/washing/dressing

Since problems of frequency and urgency in going to the toilet are prominent in MS coping with these symptoms is perhaps one of the most important topics to be discussed. One useful rule of thumb is to make sure you empty the bladder regularly, say every couple of hours or so. This won't necessarily prevent more frequent visits but it will help to keep down the risk of unexpected leaks! It will also help to keep under control the number of trips which become desperately urgent. As already mentioned, the feeling of urgency is common in MS and this is exacerbated by the physical difficulty in reaching the toilet quickly. It is crucial, therefore, to make sure that the toilet is readily accessible and a downstairs loo is clearly a 'must' in most MS homes. Placing a toilet at the top of a steep flight of stairs is like some form of medieval torture to the person with MS! To ascend the stairs at all presents a task of great difficulty; to ascend the stairs with urgency turns the task into a nightmare. As a stopgap measure portable loos such as those used by campers and caravanners can be very useful (as can pads tucked in the pants). Many MS sufferers have found, for example, that it is helpful to keep a portable toilet by the side of the bed for the first visit of the day. Stiffness in the limbs in the morning can often make even a short walk across the landing very difficult to complete comfortably at that time of the day. Similarly, a portable loo can be a boon in a house where it has not proved possible to incorporate a downstairs toilet.

Urgency or retention can occur, of course, in relation to both bladder and bowels. It is equally important, therefore, to maintain regularity in bowel movements according to the person's own pattern of regularity. With some people this may be once daily; with others more or less frequently. Constipation should be avoided if possible since in MS this often seems to have the effect of weakening bladder control. The attempt to maintain regularity is also important even when the symptoms in MS are at the opposite extreme—hesitancy, retention or difficulty in going to the toilet. There are a number of drugs available for assisting these problems and the GP should be able to advise on these.

Washing and bathing in MS can present problems. It is the claim of many MS sufferers that 'I haven't washed my feet for years'! Where the mobility of legs and arms is impaired it can often be almost impossible to reach the feet with the hands. Sometimes by sitting in a chair a person will be able to wash certain parts of the body more easily but even this approach may not always help. Similarly baths become out of the question for some people although the district nurse may be able to arrange for a 'bathing visit'. Many MS sufferers, however, whilst finding it possible to lower themselves into the bath find that climbing out afterwards (even with help) proves impossible. There are many stories about MS sufferers taking a bath on their own, letting the water out and then being unable to climb out of the bath without assistance. The window cleaner might well oblige if he were in the vicinity but one cannot always rely on his services!

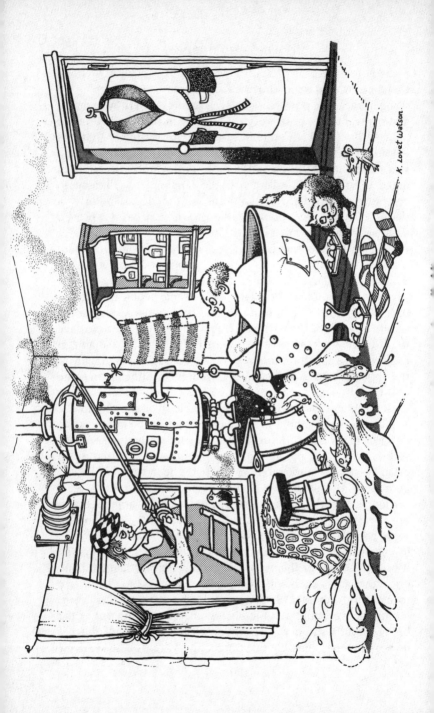

K. Lovet Watson.

The use of a bath seat (available from the local Social Services Department) is sometimes beneficial and 'grab handles' placed on the wall above the bath can be most helpful. Such handles can also be of assistance in other parts of the house (for example, toilet). Some people with MS find that they are able to use a bidet and this can also be useful in washing feet. A home visit from the Community Occupational Therapist can help the MS sufferer to decide upon and acquire the most relevant bathroom and kitchen aids. A range of aids can also be purchased privately from Boots, the chemists and charitable organisations will sometimes help with expensive items (see Chapter 6).

Perhaps the most valuable piece of washing equipment, however, as mentioned earlier, is the shower. For most people with MS a shower offers the easiest method of all-over washing. For those people who find it difficult to stand under a shower it is possible to incorporate a shower seat. The shower will enable both feet and hair to be washed. Since reaching the feet can still present a problem the long handled brushes or sponges which are available in the shops can be most useful. Similarly the problem of the 'disappearing soap' can be overcome by using 'soap on a rope'. This again is available in shops and has a loop of rope with a piece of soap on the end so that the rope can hang around the neck and soap is then readily available when required. (Some MS sufferers have found the method of hanging equipment round their necks very helpful in other respects—biros, glasses, bags in which they can carry objects from one room to another). The problem of drying oneself can be helped by using a towelling robe and some people use a hair drier or fan heater to dry their feet (but not in the bathroom, of course, where it would be electrically unsafe)!

Although the shower might help in washing hair it doesn't necessarily solve the problem of dealing with the hair at the drying and styling stages. For some MS sufferers raising the arms above shoulder level is very tiring and, especially for women, this can create considerable problems in setting their own hair. The assistance of a relative or friend in this exercise is often much appreciated. This can be a welcome social as well as functional occasion. A regular hair shampoo and set in the company of a good friend can be a marvellous tonic. Assistance from family or friends is also valuable in relation to other tasks which MS sufferers may find difficult such as finger- and toe-nail cutting and shaving. For the housebound the local authority can arrange visits from a chiropodist.

All the problems of physical immobility which apply to washing also apply to dressing. What takes five minutes for most people will take an hour for someone with MS. Putting on socks or tights can be a major operation. Some people find it useful to dress one half of the body at a time so that one sock or one leg of the tights, one leg of the pants and trousers and one shoe would be pulled on first and then the other side. Getting clothes on over the head is often a problem and, therefore, front-opening garments are a help. For women fastening a bra strap can present an awkward problem and some people seem to find that the most effective solution is to do the strap up in front and then twist the bra round. Clothes without too many buttons or fasteners are obviously important for people with MS. Velcro can replace zips and is much easier to manage. Trousers with elasticated tops are both easy to get on and to pull down when reaching the toilet. Slip-on shoes or shoes with straps are easier to get on and off than shoes with laces; or elastic shoe laces may be used. As far as nightwear is concerned some people find nightdresses or pyjamas with a slippery texture allow them to turn over in bed more easily.

Mobility

Advice about mobility depends a great deal upon the type of symptoms and their severity and the Department of Transport have prepared a most informative booklet (*Door to Door: a guide to transport for disabled people*) which covers all aspects of mobility from aids and benefits to air and sea travel. This booklet is available free from Social Security offices.

For many MS sufferers all that is required is some assistance with balance and a walking stick will frequently suffice. A child's push-chair can also be of considerable assistance in the early days of MS since this gives a valuable stability in walking. Similarly shopping trollies, providing they are well oiled and not too full, can help with walking. Another walking aid is the 'walk about'[5] which consists of a frame on wheels to which a shopping basket can be attached; a Uniscan 'A' frame walking aid with a resting seat is also a useful aid.[6]

Many people with MS are able to drive a car either normally or with adapted controls. The Mobility Allowance is available for MS sufferers and this can be used to help in the purchase of cars (a special Motability scheme is also available for this purpose) or for the payment of taxi fares or to help with transport costs in general (see Chapter 6.) Associations such as the Disabled Drivers' Association can help to keep people up to date with the variety of car conversions available. The most common are hand controls. It is also possible, however, to provide such facilities as left-foot accelerator pedals on automatic cars to aid someone with a right-sided weakness. The Banstead Place Mobility Centre will offer help and advice on choosing an appropriate car or adaptation and is equipped to provide individual assessments. (See Chapter 6.)

If someone with MS is able to drive then tasks such as going to work, shopping and collecting children from school become much easier. Local authorities supply special parking discs to help disabled drivers in parking for longer periods than able-bodied drivers and for stopping at points close to their destination (for example, outside or at the rear entrance to a food store). One of the difficulties, however, which confronts MS sufferers is that the physical effort of reaching a shopping centre can so reduce the store of energy that the shopping itself frequently needs to be greatly curtailed. Parking near to the shop becomes in these circumstances absolutely essential. It is essential also from the point of view of loading shopping into the car. Carrying heavy bags is often an impossibility and assistance may be required for loading the car. Fortunately many shops are sympathetic to the needs of disabled people in this respect.

Travelling by bus or train is something which presents difficulties for MS sufferers since both require considerable agility on entering and leaving the vehicle. British Rail and coach operators, however, do make special provision for the disabled where possible. One of the hazards of MS is that people may appear perfectly healthy and keen bus drivers sometimes shut the doors or move off before they have appreciated the degree of the passenger's disability. The use of a car is therefore likely to be more appropriate for MS sufferers, whether their own car or that of a relative or friend. Many people have found by experience that what appears at first sight to be a very comfortable car may be rather awkward when it comes to ease of access for someone who is physically handicapped. There is no substitute for trying out particular car models for yourself if you are thinking of buying one but there are one or two general points which might be of help. Most people find it helpful to enter a car by backing in! The person sits on the seat and then brings his or her legs in afterwards. In order to do this comfortably the door needs to open widely and to remain open. Although cloth upholstery is very comfortable for travelling, plastic seats may sometimes assist getting in and out of cars because the person can slide across more easily. Grab handles on the inside can also be helpful to the disabled. The boot should be sufficiently large to take a wheelchair and estate models are clearly valuable from this point of view.

If the stage comes at which someone with MS needs to resort to a wheelchair then a new set of considerations arise. Most people with MS would advise that one should 'keep out of a wheelchair as long as possible'. At some point, however, a wheelchair often becomes a necessity in order to maintain an adequate degree of mobility. The use of a wheelchair for part of the day can also serve to conserve energy for other periods when some standing or walking is necessary. To resort to a wheelchair in such circumstances is far from an admission of defeat. It is a sound and well-proven strategy by which to combat fatigue and conserve energy. Transition to wheelchair-use, however, is psychological-ly often quite difficult. In a wheelchair which requires to be pushed the person immediately becomes dependent upon the pusher and a certain degree of autonomy has to be surrendered. There is also a tendency on the part of other people to treat the person in the wheelchair as if he or she is mentally as well as physically disabled. The 'Does he take sugar?' phenomenon is very common. Well meaning people tend to ignore people in wheelchairs as individuals and talk over their heads to their companions. Nothing can be more infuriating and frustrating to the wheelchair-bound person. It is important also to realise that the wheelchair user's view of the outside world remains basically the same as that of the able-bodied except that it is a view from a seated position. Disabled people don't tend, therefore, at first to see the image of themselves as wheelchair-bound unless faced by a mirror or photograph and this image is one to which they will need time to adjust.

There are also a number of drawbacks and limitations concerning wheelchair design. One MS sufferer sums it up like this:

> If one accepts the premise that a wheelchair is a form of transport, which it is, then one can only stress how very limited is the choice and variety. While there are Boat Shows and Motor Shows that fill Earls Court exhibition hall, the variety of wheelchairs available would fill my sitting room. Babies also are far better catered for than the disabled, for them imagi-nation and innovation seems to have completely dried up. The baby, for instance, has a hood and a pram cover, the infirm have no protection against the elements whatsoever . . . The baby faces the pusher the adult has his back turned so that should he wish to stop at a certain shop not a word that he says can be heard. The baby frequently has a row of little plastic toys overhead, why could not the adult have a little plastic purse at the side for glasses and money! The pram often has a tray underneath for parcels, the wheelchair has no such device.

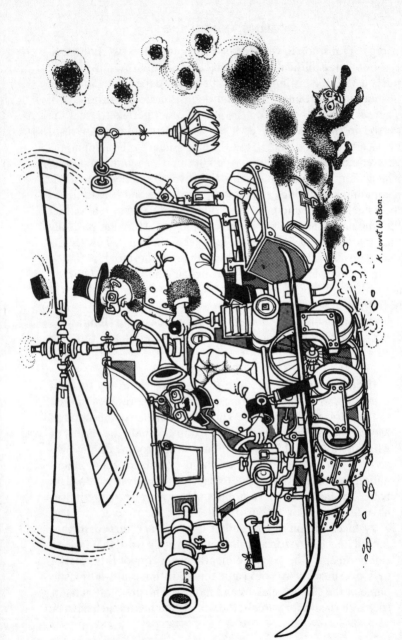

K. Lovet Watson.

There are also a number of drawbacks and limitations concerning wheelchair design . . .

A wheelchair has to have a pump; on a bicycle there is a place for it where it grips on, on a wheelchair there is nowhere to put it . . . If one could, the ideal thing would be to have two [wheelchairs], one for out-of-doors and one for indoors, the latter padded and with the same loose covers as the rest of the sitting room, that could be taken off and washed, and matching the rest of the suite so not making one stick out like a sore thumb . . . For the outdoor model there needs to be some really way-out thinking, perhaps a rickshaw type of vehicle as seen in Singapore, where the driver or escort would be alongside like a motor bike and sidecar.

For the wheelchair pusher the most important point to remember is probably the kerb drill: 'up forwards, down backwards'.

Although the variety of wheelchairs is not great there are a number of decisions which the disabled person will need to make. If a wheelchair is only required very occasionally, for example to take the person down a long approach footpath to the beach which can't be reached by car, then something like the very portable Buggy Major[7] could be a great asset. For more permanent use there are a variety of chairs available via the GP. These may be either for a helper to push or for the person to propel by use of the hands. For those people unable to use a self-propelled wheelchair then an electrically propelled version may be available. These may be also purchased privately. Some electric wheelchairs are not suitable for use both indoors and outdoors so it is necessary to check whether the model is a dual-purpose one if it is required for use both inside and outside the home.

Shopping

Shopping expeditions need to be very well planned. It is not possible to engage in the luxury of a 'shopping ramble' in which you move from shop to shop picking up an odd article here and a few bits of grocery there. In general people with MS find that they become very fatigued by such an approach. It is probably better to plan on going to one or two shops only for very specific items and to add further shopping only if the main objectives have been achieved without becoming overtired. The transport problems have been discussed in the previous section.

For many people with MS mail order firms have proved a great assistance as with the sufferer who says: 'I mainly shop by mail order, very satisfactorily. I run a catalogue, it gives me an interest and keeps my brain ticking over having to do the paper work. It brings friends to see and pay me.' Other people rely on delivery services a great deal and on the help of friends. Relatives and friends may need to help the person with MS quite often with specific tasks such as the collection of the Mobility Allowance, Post Office and banking transactions.

Holidays

In general holidays tend to be organised for the able-bodied. Many guest-houses and hotels are quite inaccessible for the disabled. Brochures frequently present the most attractive picture of a holiday residence but fail to mention that there is a steep flight of steps to the entrance! There are a limited number of places only with bedrooms and bathrooms on the ground floor and, although some hotels provide lifts these are not always sufficiently large to accommodate a wheelchair! Fortunately, there are some handbooks which give fuller information about such details—*Holidays for Disabled people* is one such book.[8] There is still need, however, for a much more comprehensive range of booklets on this topic.

Many MS families have found that self-catering holidays are successful provided that the accommodation is selected carefully. There are a number of bungalows available for hire and some specially converted holiday caravans. Occasionally branches of the MS Society will have such accommodation available for their members. (See Chapter 5.) People with MS often find travelling tiring, however, and journeys will need to be carefully planned. Holiday routes need a liberal sprinkling of loo halts, in particular. (See *Access to Public Conveniences*[9] for a useful holiday planning aid. There is also a *National Key Scheme* under which a number of toilets for the disabled throughout the UK have been fitted with special locks, keys for which may be obtained from the Local Authority or the Royal Association for Disability and Rehabilitation. A list of these toilets is available from RADAR.)

For those people who like to travel abroad the travel agencies generally supply good information about facilities for the disabled. Air and sea travel is normally quite feasible and the disabled are generally very well looked after. Individual ferry/airlines will supply details of services offered and on air travel a free booklet is available—*Care in the Air—Advice for Handicapped Passengers.*[10]

Interests

It is very important that people with MS should not cut themselves off from outside interests and social events because of their handicap. In the early stages of the disease the MS sufferer may become embarrassed at having to leave parties early or at having to explain to acquaintances who have invited them to tea that they daren't come because they haven't got a downstairs loo! For people in a wheelchair there is often a period when they feel quite embarrassed about their position. It is virtually impossible for someone in a wheelchair to slip in at the back quietly and unobserved! Most people, however, gradually come to the point where they accept that the advantages of increased mobility which a wheelchair brings far outweigh the initial disadvantages and embarrassments; but a few have to fight to reach this point of adjustment and require a good deal of support from family and friends.

Despite the difficulties people with MS often seem to manage to enter into an increasingly full social life. There are many leisure pursuits which can be engaged in despite physical handicap and new interests are often developed through being a member of the local branch of the MS Society. Many MS sufferers manage to hold down full-time or part-time jobs or run the house. Others have found time for writing, painting, photography. Television, reading and music offer accessible areas for enjoyment and entertainment. Cinemas and theatres are not always quite so accessible. Some cinemas will not accept wheelchairs and at the theatre it is often necessary to sit in a prescribed area. As one woman with MS, put it: 'If you insist on sitting in your wheelchair . . . you are obliged to sit opposite the gents.' There is, however, a helpful booklet produced by RADAR which gives details of access to cinemas and theatres.[11] As far as sport is concerned there are people with MS who enjoy swimming, riding and occasionally activities like table-tennis. Darts, chess and cards are all examples of games which people can enjoy with MS. The more strenuous aspects of gardening are often too fatiguing for someone with MS but a great deal of gardening is possible, for example greenhouse gardening, flower bed gardening (raised flower beds for the wheelchair bound) and house plants. The book *Gardening is for Everyone*[12] has some very useful suggestions for the disabled gardener.

The person with MS faces very many problems and difficulties but these can frequently be overcome or modified if tackled with a resolute spirit. MS is often said to be characterised by a certain cheerfulness of mind or euphoria and it is true that MS sufferers do seem to bear the illness with a great degree of courage and positive thinking. Most people with MS, however, would probably object to the view that this is a feeling of well-being which stems from a lack of appreciation of the serious nature of the disease. MS sufferers are quite aware of the problems and can become quite depressed in the face of them. In general, though, by regarding the disease as a challenge they seem to find renewed strength to tackle their problems and in doing so provide a tremendous example of courage and tenacity to the more able-bodies among us. Indeed people with MS often seem to live much fuller lives than able-bodied individuals and whilst coping with their immediate problems they are also hoping for the breakthrough in research which might indicate the cause of the disease and provide pointers to its cure.

The person with MS, therefore, tries to live a positive existence—an approach well illustrated by the following comments from two MS sufferers:

During my schooldays I enjoyed the normal healthy ambitions to play football and cricket for England. These ambitions have now been replaced by a more down to earth one which is to walk a straight line unassisted for fifteen yards. My main prayer is that this ambition is fulfilled as I am confident that I shall be able to build up fifteen yards to twice around the world.

I believe in the power of positive thinking—don't look at what you can't do, concentrate on the things you can do. There is usually another way of doing things . . . be flexible. Treat it as a challenge—try and plan your day—work rest work rest principle—don't let people take over completely but be happy to let them help you when you are tired. Keep going. Get your priorities right.

MS can hit hard but the MS sufferer can hit harder. It is surprising how effectively many people with MS manage to fight off the worst features of the disorder and find hidden strengths both in themselves and in members of their immediate family. It is interesting too how many MS sufferers find an amusing side to their illness. Stories told by MS sufferers themselves with a twinkle in their eye range from the married woman who trips into the arms of her milkman 'who didn't know she cared!' to the story of 'the uncontrollable leg':

In bed . . . my leg would develop a violent uncontrollable spasm which often resulted with the knee causing a heavy blow to my wife's backside. I believe the leg which at such times has a mind of its own, enjoys the experience as changing bed positions has failed to totally eliminate such occurrences.

The ability to laugh at the symptoms of the disease is a great benefit to MS sufferers.

In summary, perhaps the three most important guiding principles for coping with MS are the three Ps: be Patient, Positive and Plan ahead. With such an approach coping becomes bearable even enriching, and hoping, the forerunner of curing, keeps the spirit of optimism alive. One seventy-year-old woman who was a member of the local MS branch provides a marvellous example of this resolute spirit. She suffered from MS for thirty years and yet she kept alert and alive, looking after her ninety-year-old mother with the solicitous attention of a much younger person! Such a story must give hope to even the most faint-hearted.

5

Making New Friends Through the Multiple Sclerosis Society

Probably the majority of newly diagnosed MS sufferers have no idea of the work of the national Multiple Sclerosis Society and its branches. And frequently in the period of adjustment following the disclosure the sufferer feels a lack of desire, or even antagonism towards the idea of becoming involved with the MS Society. Cunningham[1] in her study of the self-perceived problems of a group of multiple sclerosis sufferers noted that often there was an interval of at least two years between being told the diagnosis and contacting the MS Society's Head Office for information or joining the local Branch.

This reluctance stems partly from an unwillingness of sufferers to see people at a 'club for the disabled' who are more disabled than themselves. While this attitude is so easily understood, the newly diagnosed sufferers should be reassured that if they become members of a branch they are not obliged to attend the monthly meetings. Indeed, in our branch, about one-third of the members with MS have never come to a meeting. Yet by being members of the Branch they receive regular information about development into the cause and treatment of MS, new social services or financial benefits that have been introduced and other news of national or local activities. They also have the reassurance that there is a group of people with a special interest in MS (the Branch) which will provide help should it ever be needed.

However, for many people the branch gatherings can provide valuable companionship. One member wrote:

My friends and others didn't understand how I felt and I couldn't explain. I felt odd, an outcast, embarrassed. Until by chance . . . my sister-in-law (who is a health visitor) put me in touch with the Society. I felt at ease with the people I met, they accepted me as I am, I could identify with them . . . Joining the

MS Society has been a great pleasure with a sense of 'belonging' and has given me the most useful information of all.

Another member who does not attend meetings commented that 'the main help so far has come from the MS Society'.

There are Multiple Sclerosis Societies in countries throughout the world and the Multiple Sclerosis Society of Great Britain and Northern Ireland was founded in 1953 by Richard Cave (later Sir Richard). His wife Mary had MS, and so with special encouragement from the national society in the United States of America, he launched this Society with the dual aims of sponsoring research into the cause and cure of MS and providing a service for families with a member suffering from MS. In the following years more than 350 branches have been formed until today very nearly every city or town is covered. It is primarily through the branches that the aims of the Society are fulfilled.

The Branches

It is difficult to generalise about the activities of the 350 or so branches because they are so individual. They vary in length of experience since being founded (less than one year to thirty or more years), geographical area covered, total population providing potential membership, and financial viability. It would seem though that the majority of branches have between 80 and 125 paid-up members of whom two-thirds will be suffering from multiple sclerosis. The fund-raising potential of a branch will in part depend upon the links that it has with other fund-raising bodies and charities in the local community. Clearly, some branches are immensely successful at raising money not just to be spent on research but for the purposes of welfare among their own members.

The branches vary in the emphasis they place on allocating money for research *vis-à-vis* the welfare of their own members, and this is quite permissible, for branches are autonomous in their operation. There are no instructions sent by the Society to the branches about how to manage the day-to-day affairs, or what their priorities should be regarding welfare or research. One branch may choose to take some of its members on a vacation abroad, a second would contribute the same amount of money to research. A third branch, while not being a fund raiser on such a scale, may have a very happy atmosphere with close attention being paid to the welfare needs (no matter how small) of its members. The Society will, however, intervene if a branch intends to make money directly available to a specific research project. Under the constitution all research grants must be allocated by the Society after the research proposals have been evaluated by the Society's research advisory committee.

There are some activities which each branch committee (consisting of elected members) tries to organise. Meetings are held regularly, usually with entertainment and, for members without access to cars, transport is provided. A branch might own a mini-bus (or two or more) but more often vehicles owned by social services departments or charities such as Age Concern or the Red Cross are used, as well as volunteer drivers in their own cars. These gatherings are very much family affairs, particularly the special occasions of the Christmas Party, the outings and the fund-raising events.

Assistance with holidays is the biggest welfare item for many branches but it rather depends on the level of support provided by the local social services department. Again, some branches have their own holiday facilities. For example, our branch owns a five-berth caravan on a holiday camp site and it is available at subsidised rates to all families of MS sufferers. There are numerous other ways that assistance is given to members such as help with heating and with personal mobility. But perhaps the most important welfare role of the branch committee is listening to members' needs and then liaising with the agency which they think will best be able to help. It could be the social services department, the social security office, the national health service through the member's general practitioner, or a local charity known to have special welfare projects. An amazing amount has often been achieved by a carefully written letter on branch notepaper.

MS Crack

Early in 1976 MS Crack, the brainchild of Mrs Nicole Davoud, was launched. It is the 'young arm' of the Multiple Sclerosis Society and is really intended for people young in heart, who would prefer to meet in small groups in each other's homes or the pub or wherever. It is very much a self-help movement and almost one-third of the MS branches now have an MS Crack group. The newly diagnosed person may well prefer to make contact with such a group rather than with the local branch, because of its greater informality.

The Multiple Sclerosis Society of Great Britain and Northern Ireland

Around 1976 the structure of the Society was changed to allow all branches a greater opportunity of being represented on the Council, the governing body of the Society. Thus the 350 or so branches are zoned according to geographical area into nineteen associations which usually hold meetings twice yearly to exchange ideas on the management of branch affairs. Every association can elect one member (or two members if there are twenty or more branches in the association) to the Council. These are annual elections. Also two representatives of MS Crack and one from the Central Fund Raising Committee serve as Council members. In addition, six persons are elected to the Council at the Society's annual general meeting (AGM) for a three-year term of office. In the association's elections each branch has one vote, but at the AGM the total votes of a branch correspond to its paid-up membership. So the Council consists of about forty persons and responsible to it are the permanent staff at the headquarters in Effie Road, Fulham. There are six advisory committees: a Finance Advisory Committee, the Fund Raising Committee; the Medical Research Advisory Committee; MS Crack Advisory Committee, a Homes Committee and the Welfare Committee. There is also an Executive Committee responsible for the day-to-day matters of the Society.

The Society has various sources of income apart from the donations from the branches which are usually for research purposes. These sources include subscriptions, profits from sales and functions, legacies and covenants and the total amount raised each year is considerable. In 1984 the Society was twenty-ninth in the league table of voluntary income attracted by all charities. It was also one of the ten charities to which people would be most likely to give their support.[2] However, the outgoings are considerable.

Research is a priority and guidance on grant-giving is offered to the Society's Council by the Medical Research Advisory Committee. Serving on this committee are eminent medical doctors and scientists from various fields—neurology, virology, immunology, biochemistry and pathology. All research proposals are closely scrutinised and when grants are made the researchers have to report annually to the Advisory Committee. This committee has another important function. It looks carefully at all reports about new treatments claiming to improve or cure sufferers of multiple sclerosis. It then advises the Society on the information that should be circulated to the Society's members. As well as awarding research grants from its own budget, the Society administers two other research funds: the Jacqueline du Pré Multiple Sclerosis Research Fund and the Stuart Henry Multiple Sclerosis Research Fund.

On the welfare side, the Society either owns or has considerable investments in at least six holiday or short-stay homes for multiple sclerosis sufferers. Helen Ley House in Leamington Spa, Warwickshire is the Society's short-stay home and the holiday homes include the Richard Cave Home just outside North Berwick, East Lothian; Holmhill in Grantown on Spey, Morayshire; Peter Scott Martin House in Ballymena, County Antrim; Orcombeleigh in Exmouth, Devon; and Kenninghall in Worthing, West Sussex. In addition to these homes the Society has two hotels, the Brambles Respite Care Hotel at Horley in

Surrey and the Danygraig Respite Care Hotel at Porthcawl in South Glamorganshire. As these homes and hotels are costly to run, the weekly rates for guests are heavily subsidised (up to one-half) by the Society.

Another greatly valued welfare activity is the counselling service provided by the Head Office through the Welfare Secretaries. As well as liaising with branches and MS Crack groups about welfare matters, they answer dozens of calls daily from individuals seeking advice on many topics. They can also offer practical assistance in cases where the local branch has been unable to cope.

But it is the Society's information service which reaches out to all members and this is masterminded by the General Secretary. The service operates in three ways. The first is keeping in touch with all developments relevant to the MS Society as a whole (for example, progress in research, new government decisions affecting the disabled, new ways of raising funds, cooperation between international MS societies) and reporting to the branches. A branch secretary receives a package of documents monthly. The second activity is the direct liaison between the Head Office of the Society and individual branches especially those being newly founded, MS Crack groups, and associations, and this frequently means visits all over the country for the General Secretary and other members of the head office staff.

The Society's publications are its third source of information. The magazine *MS News* is supplied free of charge to all paid-up members of the Society—46,000 copies are now being printed of each issue and the total readership is thought to exceed 120,000 persons. In response to readers' overwhelming requests for news about MS research, each issue contains special research reports or interviews with research clinicians and scientists. Readers' own letters and articles appear as well as special articles on such topics as mobility, employment opportunities and holidays. Also covered regularly are welfare matters, the MS Crack movement, overseas news, any policy decisions taken by Council, major fund-raising events organised by the Fund Raising Committee or by the Jacqueline du Pré or Stuart Henry research funds, and news supplied by local branches.

The *MSS Bulletin* is also produced by the Society. This monthly bulletin of about fifteen pages covers many topics; for example, any new government benefits, new schemes or events being arranged by the Society, the MS Crack movement, holiday information and a For Sale column. One special feature is its coverage of the developments in other charities and helpful organisations of which MS sufferers can take advantage. At the moment the *MSS Bulletin* is sent to some members of the branch committees with the idea that information will be extracted from the bulletin and included in the Branch's own newsletters. However, as the bulletin covers such a wide range of interests, only a certain amount will get into the local newsletters and individual members may receive their own copies by applying to Head Office. A small annual charge is made for the bulletin.

The company Securicor Ltd has donated its services to distributing much of the information prepared by the society. All the *MS News* are boxed and transported to the branch committees who distribute them locally. Again, Securicor deliver the packages sent by Head Office to the branch secretaries, and the company's branches will help out with transport difficulties experienced by an MS Branch.

So, how do people (sufferers, their family and friends, or anyone else) become members of the Multiple Sclerosis Society? If local branch members are not already known, the easiest thing is to contact the head office of the Society who will supply the address of the local branch secretary. The subscription to the Society is very small and it is paid direct to a Branch. The address of the Society is: The Multiple Sclerosis Society of Great Britain and Northern Ireland, 25 Effie Road, Fulham, London SW6 1EE. Tel. 01-736 6267.

6

Other Sources of Practical Help
Outside the Family

The purpose of this book has been to show how it is possible to come to terms with, and cope with, a disability. For many MS sufferers the great challenge is to retain their independence but, as Chapter 4 suggests, in doing so there is an in-built contradiction in terms—namely, that in order best to retain that precious independence, the sufferer must be willing and able to make use of the very many areas of practical help which exist outside the immediate family and friends. In general, the most successful adjustment is made by thinking out the problems involved in leading the kind of life which you want to lead, and then looking for solutions. Of all the problems, probably the most common and frustrating to the disabled is that of fatigue, and therefore the most important initial solution to be found is that of discovering easier and less tiring ways of doing the essential everyday things, so that energy and resources may be saved for doing those things which, from personal choice, make life most worthwhile.

To overcome a practical problem, different people need different levels and forms of assistance. Aids are not necessarily the solution to every problem, and the individual may often be reluctant to accept the necessity for such an aid, feeling that its use is an admission of some sort of defeat. However, many people have found that the use of appropriate aids entirely change a life-style, and it is often true that the simplest aid is the best. We cannot hope to give detailed specialist advice on the range of equipment and the various forms of financial and practical assistance available. This chapter, however, points the reader to the sources from which specialised help and advice is available. Also included are the addresses of agencies which exist to enable the disabled person to continue to be active in special hobbies, or find new ones to develop, thus filling the need for opening up new horizons and making new friends. Finally, a list of some helpful reference books is provided to supplement those included in the main body of the text.

First points of contact

The General Practitioner

The very first point of contact will in most cases be the person's General Practitioner. Many benefits from the Social Services Department depend on the referral or recommendation of GPs, so they should be kept acquainted with any changes in the condition of the patient. The GP can make arrangements for the disabled person to be contacted regarding such essential assistance as Home Helps, the Health Visitor, the District Nurse, and either the GP or the hospital consultant can arrange for the loan of aids such as wheelchairs or walking sticks. Wheelchairs can also be obtained on short-term loan from agencies such as the Red Cross Society. Many disabled people will receive regular visits from the District Nurse, although the regularity of such visits will obviously depend upon the nature of the person's condition. Medical aid which might include hospital treatment, or home physiotherapy or chiropody can also be arranged through liaison between the GP and the Medical Social Worker (a social worker attached to a hospital).

Hospital

The MS sufferer may be referred to the Physical Medicine Department for an assessment of needs in relation to mobility and daily living. Walking aids such as sticks, crutches and walking frames may be provided on loan from the physiotherapy department, and arrangements can be made via the nearest Department of Health and Social Security appliance centre to borrow a wheelchair. Physiotherapy and hydrotherapy might be recommended and the Occupational Therapist asked to carry out the assessment of daily needs on such matters as kitchen and bathroom facilities. Arrangements will be made for the provision of appropriate aids and adaptations to the home.

The Social Services Department

The Chronically Sick and Disabled Persons' Act (1970) gave details of some of the services that should be available to the disabled, and required local authorities to identify the disabled in their areas and to provide information of the services available to them. However, it appears that not all authorities have been successful in compiling a Register of the Disabled, and it is often unclear whether the disabled person receives attention from a Social Worker as a result of being registered, or whether the process works in reverse. It therefore seems advisable for disabled people themselves to take steps to become registered. Contact with the Social Services will normally begin with a visit from the Local Authority Social Worker or Community Occupational Therapist. But whether or not such contact has been made, information and advice about a number of services is available through the staff of the Social Service Department who liaise with other departments. The services may vary slightly between different authorities but they will probably include the following:

(a) Practical assistance in the home, including provision or loan of special aids and structural alterations to assist mobility about the home and independence in general.

(b) Structural alterations to homes, such as the widening of doors and construction of ramps, as well as the provision of walking aids and aids for bathroom and kitchen; also such major items as hydraulic hoists and adjustable tilting beds can all be grant assisted or provided by local authorities. Electronic support systems such as POSSUM are also available, and severely disabled patients are advised to make enquiries about these, since evidence suggests that many people who could use them to their advantage know little or nothing about them.

(c) Help from Occupational Therapists and Physiotherapists may sometimes be available via the Social Services Department as well as the hospital. They can be contacted through the GP or Social Worker. The Occupational Therapist assesses the practical needs of disabled people to live and work as normally as possible, operating on a visiting basis and giving advice on equipment and necessary alterations; the physiotherapist helps to maintain bodily movement as far as possible, and will in some cases make regular home visits.

(d) Recreational and educational facilities: these vary among authorities, but many provide Day Centres and can give information on special courses, adult education centres and other facilities provided by voluntary organisations.

(e) Assistance with the provision of telephones for those who are at risk or isolated from friends and neighbours— information is also available from British Telecom on special adaptations for the disabled, particularly the hard of hearing.

(f) Provision of television and radio for those isolated from social contact.

(g) Home Help Service: this can be provided for as little or as much time per week as is thought necessary, and the cost of this help with housework, cooking and shopping is based on a means test assessment.

(h) Holidays: a number of special publications exist dealing with holidays for the disabled (see, for example, *Holidays for Disabled People*[1]) and local authorities can give financial assistance in providing holidays.

(i) Parking discs: most authorities provide special badges enabling more convenient parking for the disabled.

(j) Attendance at and help in getting to Day Centres, Luncheon Clubs and Social Clubs—these are often run by voluntary organisations, but the Social Worker can put you in contact with them.

(k) Meals on Wheels—provision of meals can be provided by the Social Services Department on direct application.

(l) Housing: although local authorities have limited resources for the housing of the disabled, many people can be moved to housing more suitable for their needs and some authorities provide purpose-built houses and flats. In general rehousing is indicated where access to the bathroom or toilet is difficult, or where it is necessary for a person to be housed on one floor level.

(m) Home chiropody treatment is sometimes available.

Disablement Resettlement Officer

Disablement Resettlement Officers work from local employment offices or Jobcentres helping to operate the quota scheme whereby employers with twenty or more employees are required to employ at least 3 per cent disabled persons. They are specially trained to help disabled people to resettle into suitable employment, and have close contact with employers, doctors, hospital and social services. Their aim is to help disabled people to achieve their maximum potential for employment, and they can be a source of practical help and morale boosting for the newly diagnosed sufferer who can see little or no working future ahead.

Benefits and allowances

For most of us the complicated range of benefits and allowances available is a frightening maze and many people, rather than become lost in its bureaucratic intricacies or face possible disappointment, will do without. There are, however, many benefits which can considerably help to improve the quality of life for the disabled person and his/her family. Leaflets and advice can be obtained from any local Social Security office, and particularly helpful are the leaflets entitled 'Which Benefit?' (FB2) and 'Social Security Benefit Rates' (NI 196). You can also call the Social Security Freephone on 0800 666 555 (in England, Scotland and Wales) or 0800 616 7571 (in Northern Ireland) for general information about benefits. There are also two other very important sources of information for discovering what current benefits are available, who is eligible for them and how to set about obtaining them:

1. The Disability Rights Handbook

Published by: The Disability Alliance ERA,
                 25, Denmark Street, LONDON WC2H 8NJ
                 Tel. 01-240 0806

This is an annual publication, updated in April of each year, and is a fully comprehensive guidebook to rights, benefits and services available to disabled people and their families, making it easy to discover which benefits you are entitled to, and showing clearly the procedure for obtaining them.

2. Disablement Information and Advice Lines (DIAL) UK

Head Office: DIAL (UK), Dial House,
                117 High Street, Clay Cross,
                CHESTERFIELD, Derbyshire
                Tel. 0246 250055

This is a nationwide telephone information and advice service, manned by trained disabled volunteers, and able to give thorough up-to-date advice and information on benefits, allowances and services. There are over 100 local DIAL offices throughout the UK, whose telephone numbers can be found in local newspapers, Access Guides, telephone directories, through Directory Enquiries (192), or by application to the Head Office.

Enquiries to the local Social Security office may be necessary in order to check on the availability of benefits in individual cases, but the main benefits are as follows:

(a)   Attendance allowance: this is a tax-free, non contributory benefit available to people who are severely disabled and who have needed looking after day and/or night for at least six months. (Further information is given in leaflet NI 205 from a Social Security Office.)

(b) Invalid Care Allowance: a non-contributory allowance for men and single women of working age who have to stay at home to care for a severely disabled relative who is getting attendance allowance. The allowance is liable to tax (Leaflet NI 212).

(c) Mobility Allowance: a tax-free, non-contributory allowance for people below retirement age who are unable, or nearly unable to walk (Leaflet NI 211).

(d) Assistance with fares to work: for severely disabled persons who are registered as disabled, and who, for reasons of their disability, are unable to use the public transport for all or part of their journey to and from work, resulting in extra travel costs. Claims should be made through the Disablement Resettlement Officer at the Jobcentre (Leaflet PWD 1).

(e) Family Credit: this is a means-tested Social Security benefit for families on low wages who have children (Leaflet NI 261 'A guide to family credit').

(f) Free dental treatment, free prescriptions, vouchers for glasses: families or people on low incomes or receiving income support and some disabled people may be eligible for assistance. For full details check in the *Disability Rights Handbook*.

(g) Housing Benefit: this is a means-tested benefit which gives help with paying rent and/or general rates to people on low incomes. Disabled people may also be entitled to rate rebates by virtue of having facilities such as central heating, a garage, an extra toilet or bathroom, which are necessitated by their disability. (Leaflet RR on housing benefit from the Citizens' Advice Bureau or Department of the Environment.)

(h) Income Support (IS): this is a means-tested benefit for people on low incomes. Extra financial help may also be available in certain circumstances through the discretionary Social Fund. Check with your local Social Security office for details.

(i) Invalidity Benefit: this is available for people who have been receiving sickness benefit for over twenty-eight weeks and for people who become chronically ill before reaching retirement age (Leaflet NI 16A).

(j) Severe Disablement Allowance: this is a weekly cash benefit, tax-free and non-means tested, for people who have been unable to work for at least twenty-eight weeks but who do not have sufficient National Insurance contributions to qualify for sickness and invalidity benefit. It cannot normally be paid for the first time after the pensionable age. The regulations relating to this allowance are rather complicated, and it is advisable either to consult your local Social Security office (Leaflet NI 252), or look at the comprehensive information given in the *Disability Rights Handbook*

(k) Hospital Patients' travelling expenses: this is available to both in-patients and out-patients, and although it is always available for those receiving family credit or income support, it can often apply to others on a fairly low income, and may cover the expenses of a friend or relative if an escort is needed (Leaflet H 11 from a hospital).

(l) Tax allowances: these are described in the PAYE Coding Guide which comes with an income tax form, or is available from any Inland Revenue Office. Disabled people may be entitled to allowances such as the additional personal allowance for children where a wife is incapacitated, or to the daughter's service allowance where a daughter is caring for a parent.

(m) Motability: this is a voluntary organisation which can help you to use your mobility allowance to obtain a car or electric wheelchair on terms better than you might otherwise achieve. A leaflet entitled 'Introducing Motability' is available from Social Security offices, and explains the scheme in detail.

Four key organisations

The Multiple Sclerosis Society

Headquarters: 25 Effie Road, Fulham,
London SW6 1EE — Tel. 01-736 6267

Much of the work of the Society and its branches has been described in Chapter 5, but it should be emphasised that for the MS sufferer the Society can offer much assistance on a variety of problems. Local branches can help through links with the Social Services, advice, financial and practical help, and simply through contact with others who have faced or are facing the same problems. The details of local branches can be obtained from your local library, a Citizen's Advice Bureau, or often in local newspapers.

The Disabled Living Foundation

380/384 Harrow Road, London W9 2HU
Tel. 01-289 6111

The DFL provides a really valuable information service for the disabled and an aids centre. The information service can supply up-to-date information about manufacturers, stockists and prices of aids, whilst at the aids centre professional help and advice can be given, although it is wise to make an appointment in order to ensure that one of the advisers is available to help you.

The Disability Alliance ERA

25 Denmark Street, London WC2H 8NJ
Tel. 01-240 0806

This is a federation of sixty organisations of or for disabled people, with the aim of introducing a comprehensive approach to financing disability, and restructuring the existing methods of social security benefits. It publishes research reports on specific problems of disability and a *Handbook* encouraging the taking up of existing benefits, as well as running a *Welfare Rights Information Service*.

The Royal Association for Disability and Rehabilitation (RADAR)

25 Mortimer Street,
London W1N 8AB
Tel. 01-637 5400

The importance of this organisation can hardly be over-emphasised. It provides an information service about manufacturers and stockists of aids and, on receipt of enquiries explaining a problem in full, will attempt to give comprehensive information and advice free of charge. Its broadsheets of information on such subjects as transport, wheelchairs and holidays are up to date and comprehensive and are well worth acquiring if you are contemplating personal expenditure on aids or equipment. The Association also has a permanent display of a range of aids for the disabled, and this is staffed by physiotherapists and occupational therapists. The NAIDEX CONFERENCE AND EXHIBITION is another excellent exhibition of aids and equipment held twice a year, and all information on this can be obtained from the RADAR Head Office.

Other agencies

The Aid Centre

182 Brighton Road, Coulsdon, Surrey CR3 2NF
Tel. 01-645 9014

Offers professional advice on all aspects of buying a car, new or second hand, vehicle finance and necessary adaptations.

Age Concern England (National Old People's Welfare Council)

Bernard Sunley House, 60 Pitcairn Road,
Mitcham, Surrey CR4 3LL
Tel. 01-640 5431

Although concerned with the welfare and rights of the aged, local branches often hire out vehicles to other organisations and can solve problems of transport for local MS branches.

ARMS (Action Research into Multiple Sclerosis)

4a Chapel Hill, Stanstead, Essex CM24 8AG
Tel. 0279 815553

A self-help organisation seeking to encourage research and education on MS. There is a twenty-four-hour counselling service operated from 01-222 3123 (London), 021-476 4229 (Birmingham) or 041-945 3939 (Glasgow).

Association of Disabled Professionals

The Stables, 73 Pound Road,
Banstead, Surrey SM7 2HU
Tel. 073 73 52366

This is a self-help group seeking to improve the rehabilitation of disabled people. It publishes a quarterly Newsletter and a House Bulletin.

Banstead Place Mobility Centre

Park Road, Banstead,
Surrey SM7 3EE
Tel. 073 7351674

Offers information and advice on any outdoor mobility problems including the provision of individual assessments and trial/ demonstration facilities in relation to the choice of appropriate adaptions on wheelchair models. Enquiries should be made in writing to the Mobility Office.

British Computer Society

13 Mansfield Street, London W1M 0BP
Tel. 01-637 0471

A specialist group which will offer specific advice on activities relating to computing and the disabled.

British Red Cross Society

9 Grosvenor Crescent, London SW1X 7EJ
Tel. 01-235 5454

Can often be helpful in solving problems of a practical nature, particularly with regard to transport or wheelchairs.

British Sports Association for the Disabled

Hayward House, Barnard Crescent,
Aylesbury, Bucks HP21 9PP
Tel. 0926 27889

The recognised governing body for all types of sports for the disabled, obtaining grants for disabled sports and organising international sporting events.

Central Bureau for Educational Visits and Exchanges

Seymour Mews House, Seymour Mews,
London W1H 9PE
Tel. 01-486 5101

Will supply advice and suitable contacts to groups and individuals wishing to make educational visits and exchanges.

College of Speech Therapists

Harold Poster House, 6 Lechmere Road,
London NW2 5BU
Tel. 01-459 8521

Provides a number of pamphlets on remedial speech therapy and will advise on the location of qualified speech therapists.

Disability Alliance ERA (see page 66)

Disabled Christians' Fellowship

50, Clare Road, Kingswood, Bristol BS15 1PJ
Tel. 0272 616141

Publishes a monthly newsletter which can be sent free of charge to any disabled person throughout the British Isles and overseas. Tapes and cassettes are also available on free loan, and great emphasis is placed upon linking members through correspondence, exchange of cassettes and by telephone. There are many local branches, and holidays are organised each year.

Disabled Drivers' Association

Ashwellthorpe Hall, Ashwellthorpe,
Norwich NR16 1EX
Tel. 050 841 449

The organisation will help and advise disabled people on all matters of mobility. An annual subscription entitles members to receive its magazine.

Disabled Drivers' Motor Club

Cosy Nook, Cottingham Way,
Thrapston, Northants NN14 4PL
Tel. 0801 24724

Gives help and advice to the disabled motorist, and the annual subscription entitles members to the bi-monthly magazine.

Disablement Income Group and Charitable Trust

Attlee House, Toynbee Hall,
28 Commercial Street, London E1 6LR
Tel. 01-247 2128
and
152 Morrison Street, Edinburgh EH 8BY
Tel. 031 228 1666

Aims to improve the financial situation of the disabled; the group runs an advisory service, publishes research papers and an ABC of service and information for disabled people.

Disabled Living Foundation (see page 66)

Gingerbread

35 Wellington Street, London WC2
Tel. 01-240 0953

An association with over 370 local groups seeking to encourage and promote the interests of people who, for whatever reasons, have to support or care for their families alone. Group meetings are held and advisory literature is available.

Greater London Association for the Disabled

8 Tankerton Mews Whitstable, Kent CT5 2DB
Tel. 0227 274 010

This publishes a directory of clubs in London for physically disabled people, a quarterly magazine and other specialist publications, and aims to be a source of information on local and national welfare legislation, and to press for improvements in the quality of life for disabled Londoners.

Help the Aged

St James Walk, London EC1R 0BE
Tel. 01-253 0253

Promotes day centres, hospitals and rehabilitation centres for the elderly, including the disabled, and can be helpful with transport problems.

Holiday Care Service

2 Old Bank Chambers, Station Road,
Horley, Surrey RH6 9HW
Tel. 0293 774535

Will give advice and information about agencies to contact when arranging holidays for the disabled.

Information Service for Disabled People

Northern Ireland Committee for the Handicapped,
2 Annadale Avenue, Belfast BT7 3JH
Tel. 0232 649555

Invalids at Home Trust

17 Lapstone Gardens, Kenton,
Harrow, HA3 0EB
Tel. 01-907 1706

Provides money for equipment to help invalids to live at home.

Jewish Welfare Board

221 Golders Green Road, London NW11 9DW
Tel. 01-458 3282

Jewish voluntary organisation covering Greater London, the Home Counties and the south of England, and cooperating with other voluntary organisations to meet all kinds of welfare problems for members of the Jewish community.

John Grooms Association for the Disabled

10 Gloucester Drive, London N4 2LP
Tel. 01-802 7272

Provides care and accommodation for severely disabled people, running holiday hotels, self-catering holiday units, and through a housing association promotes the provision of purpose-built flats for the disabled.

Leonard Cheshire Foundation

26-29 Maunsel Street, London SW1P 2QN
Tel. 01-828 1822

Provides residential accommodation and a wide range of activities for the severely disabled, and some holiday accommodation.

Motability

2nd Floor, Gate house, Westgate
Harlow, Essex CM20 1HR
Tel. 0279 635666

An organisation to ensure that disabled people who wish to obtain a vehicle or electric wheelchair using their mobility allowance can do so, getting the maximum value for money.

Multiple Sclerosis Society (see page 66)

National Council for Carers and their Elderly Dependants

29 Chilworth Mews, London W2 3RG
Tel. 01-742 7776

Assists single people who have infirm or disabled dependants, running an advisory service and publishing a bi-monthly newsletter.

National Council for Voluntary Organisations

26 Bedford Square, London WC1B 3HU
Tel. 01-636 4066

Issues helpful booklets on many subjects, including an annual directory called *Voluntary Agencies*, which appears in November and lists all kinds of relevant organisations, with a brief description of the work of each.

Patients Association

Room 33, 18 Charing Cross Road,
London WC2H 0HR
Tel. 01-240 0671

An independant advisory service for patients, aiming to represent and further their interests, and campaigning for improvements in the NHS. It produces a number of leaflets, for example on rights of patients, changing one's doctor, etc.

PHAB (Physically handicapped and Able-bodied)

Tavistock House North, Tavistock Square,
London WC1H 9HX
Tel. 01-388 1963

The organisation has the objective of integrating physically handicapped and able-bodied young people through leisure and social activities. Over 200 clubs meet regularly to share a variety of interests and activities, and some thirty-five holiday residential courses are held each year in Britain and abroad.

Photography for the Disabled

190 Secrett House, Ham Close,
Ham, Richmond, Surrey TW10 7PE
Tel. 01-948 2342

A registered charity providing advice, instruction and equipment for the disabled person, so that he may enjoy the recreational activity afforded by the medium of photography.

SEQUAL (formerly The Possum Users' Association)

Ddol Hir, Glyn Ceiriog, Llangollen, Clwyd
Tel. 0691 72 331

The aim of the association is to assist those very severely disabled people who rely on the electronic POSSUM Aid, and it is dedicated to the social and financial improvement of conditions for its members and the disabled in general.

Riding for the Disabled Association

Avenue R, National Agricultural Centre, Kenilworth,
Warwickshire CV8 2LY
Tel. 0203 696510

There are about 450 groups throughout the UK, each consisting of an organiser, secretary, riding instructor, usually a physiotherapist and other helpers. Riding is usually free but where schools are concerned, and individuals can afford it, contributions are welcomed. The book *Riding for the Disabled* is available from the Association.

Royal Association for Disability and Rehabilitation (see page 67)

Queen Elizabeth's Foundation for the Disabled

Leatherhead, Surrey KT22 0BN
Tel. 0372 842204

Comprises four units which provide assessment, further education, vocational training, residential sheltered work, holidays and convalescence for many hundreds of disabled people.

Scottish Information Service for the Disabled

Scottish Council on Disability, Princes House,
5 Shandwick Place, Edinburgh EH2 4RG
Tel. 031 556 3882

SPOD Sexual Problems of the Disabled

286 Camden Road, London N7 0BJ
Tel. 01-607 8851/2

Provides general information and advice in leaflet and letter form.

Womens' Royal Voluntary Service

234-244 Stockwell Road,
London SW9 9SP
Tel. 01-499 6040

About 1,500 branches exist nationwide, providing valuable social help of all kinds to the elderly and disabled.

NB. In addition to all the organisations mentioned, there are often other local groups which are prepared to give assistance in various ways, and these include the scout and guide movements, the Voluntary Bureaux, the Lions, Rotary Club and Round Table and other such organisations—the golden rule, basically, is don't be afraid to *ask*.

Some helpful reference books

AA Guide for the Disabled

The Automobile Association
Fanum House, Basingstoke
Hampshire RG21 2EA

Access Guides

Royal Association for Disability and Rehabilitation
(RADAR), 25 Mortimer Street, London W1N 8AB

There are a range of Access publications produced by RADAR covering such topics as Theatres, Cinemas, Nature Reserves, London Underground Stations, Public Conveniences, cities and towns. Many towns and cities also have their own Access Guides available from Council Offices.

An ABC of Service and General Information for Disabled People

Disablement Income Group, Toynbee Hall,
28 Commercial Street, London E1 6LR

Coping with Disablement

Consumers Association,
14 Buckingham Street, London WC2N 6DS

The Disability Rights Handbook (see page 67)

The Disability Alliance ERA
25 Denmark Street, London WC2H 8NJ

OTHER SOURCES OF PRACTICAL HELP OUTSIDE THE FAMILY

Designing for the Disabled
(by Selwyn Goldsmith)

Royal Institute of British Architects,
Publications Ltd,
66 Portland Place, London W1N 4AD

Directory for Disabled People
(by Ann Darnbrough and Derek Kinrade)

Woodhead Faulkner in association with Royal Association for
Disability and Rehabilitation (RADAR)

The New Source Book for the Disabled
(edited by Glorya Hale)

Heinemann, London

Voluntary Social Services

National Council for Social Services,
26, Bedford Square,
London WC1B 3HU

Notes

Chapter 1

1 See, for example, Matthews, W.B. (1985) *Multiple Sclerosis: The Facts*, 2nd edn (Oxford University Press) and Bauer, H.J. (1977) *A Manual on Multiple Sclerosis* (The International Federation of MS Societies). Also see the following articles: Burnfield, A. and Burnfield, P. (1978) 'Common Psychological Problems in Multiple Sclerosis', *British Medical Journal*, 1, 1193-4. (This article is reproduced in *MS News*, No. 97, Autumn 1978.) Tallis, R.C. (1981) 'Multiple Sclerosis: Diagnosing MS and telling the patient', *MS News*, No. 107, Spring.

Chapter 2

1   Many sources were consulted when writing this chapter, the main ones being: Matthews, W.B. (1985) *Multiple Sclerosis: The Facts*; and Matthews, W.B. *et al*. (1985) *McAlpine's Multiple Sclerosis*, Edinburgh, Churchill Livingstone.

2   Office of Population Censuses and Surveys (1974) *Morbidity Statistics from General Practice. Second National Study 1970-71*. Studies on Medical and Population Subjects, No. 26, London, HMSO.

3   Williams, E.S. and McKeran, R.O. (1986) 'Prevalance of Multiple Sclerosis in a South London Borough', *British Medical Journal*, 293, pp. 237-9.

4   McDonald, W. I. (1978) *MS News*, No. 98, Winter, pp. 9-16.

5   Mims, C. (1983) *MS News*, No. 117, Autumn, pp. 7-11.

6   Wiles, C. M. *et al*. (1986) 'Hyperbaric oxygen in Multiple Sclerosis: a double blind trial.' *British Medical Journal*, 292, pp. 367-71.

Chapter 3

1   *Forum* (1975) includes articles on MS—The basic facts; How to fight back; To get married or not; To have children or not; What to tell the children. From MS Society, 25 Effie Road, Fulham, London SW6 1EE.

SPOD (Sexual Problems of the Disabled), 286 Camden Road, London N7 0BJ.

Chapter 4

1   Burnfield, A. and Burnfield, P. (1978) (see note 1, Cn. 1 above).

2   A useful organisation is *Yoga for Health Foundation*, Ickwell Bury, Northill, Biggleswade, Bedfordshire SG18 9ES. Tel. 076 727271. Arranges special MS weekends.

3   From Cunningham, D.J. (1977) *Stigma and Social Isolation: self-perceived problems of a group of Multiple Sclerosis sufferers*. Health Services Research Unit, University of Kent at Canterbury.

4   AID-call Ltd, Moreton House, Moreton Hampstead, Devon TQ13 8NF. Tel. 0647 40804.

5   Obtained from Midlands Engineering Tools Co., P.O. Box 163, Breaston, Derby DE7 3UN. Tel. 03317 2510.

6   Available from Uniscan Ltd, Samson House, Arterial Road, Laindon, Essex SS15 6DR. Tel. 0268 419288.

7   The Buggy Major is available from Andrew Mclaren Ltd, Station Works, Long Buckby, Northampton NN6 7PF. Tel. 0327 842662.

8   *Holidays for Disabled People* is published by RADAR, 25 Mortimer Street, London W1N 8AB.

9   *Access to Public Conveniences* is published by RADAR (see note 8 above).

10 *Care in the air—Advice for Handicapped Passengers*. From Air Transport Users Committee, 129 Kingsway, London WC2B 6NN.

11 *Theatres and Cinemas—An Access Guide for Disabled People (England, Scotland And Wales)*. From RADAR (See note 8 above).

12 Underhill, C. and Cloet, A. *Gardening is for All*, Souvenir Press.

Chapter 5

1 Cunningham, D.J. (1977) (see note 3, Ch. 4 above).

2 Editorial (1984) *MS News*, No. 122, Winter.

Chapter 6

1 For full reference see note 8, Ch. 4 above.

Index